AF885035

# Collin Gow, C.N.C.

## Collected Works on Health and Nutrition, Volume 2 (2021–2022)

Collin Gow, C.N.C.

**With special gratitude and appreciation, I want to thank:**

**Victor of Abby's Health and Nutrition**, my clients, customers, and patrons, as well as N. Meister, Janet Guess, and all my peers within my world, past and present, for their influence, attention, care, and/or support. Thank you.

Copyright © 2022 by Collin Gow, C.N.C.

All rights reserved. This book or any portion thereof
may not be reproduced, transmitted, or used in any manner
without the express written permission of the publisher,
Naturotheology Publishing, except as permitted by U.S. copyright law.
For permissions contact:

naturotheology@protonmail.com or collingowcnc@gmail.com or go to
www.collingowcnc.wixsite.com/collingowcnc or
www.collingowcnc.com (under construction as of 1/25/2022)

# Contents

**DISCLAIMER:**

The contents of this book are not an attempt to treat, diagnose, prevent, or cure any disease or condition. Talk to your doctor before making any changes.

# Cooking Food

# Collin Gow, C.N.C.'s Cooking Principles (How to Cook & Prepare Food)

Collin Gow, C.N.C.

1/9/22

1. **Don't Cook**. The best way to cook is to not cook at all. One should strive to eat at least 51% of their foods raw. Low temperature is better than high temperature, if you do cook a food.
2. **Wet Heat**. Wet heat cooking is the second best way to cook. It consists of boiling, steaming, braising, stewing, poaching, simmering, blanching, steeping, pressure cooking, and en papillote. This method of cooking reduces advanced glycation end products, which can cause aging and inflammation and increase the risk of diabetes, cardiovascular disease, and cancer.
3. **Stainless Steel pans and pots**. Healthier than cooking with non-stick pans, which often contain a fluorine-based coating.
4. **Earthenware clay pots**. Many cultures around the world have traditionally cooked in clay pots.
5. **Wooden cooking utensils and cutting board**. Wood is healthier and more natural than plastic. Non-toxic, wild-harvested, end grain cut, non-mineral-oil-finished maple, walnut, cherry, or teak are ideal for cutting boards. Maple is the best.
6. **Cast iron pan**. Iron deficiency is the #1 most common nutrient deficiency in the world. It is #2 in the U.S..
7. **Copper pot**. Copper is antimicrobial (antiviral, antifungal, and antibacterial) and necessary for collagen synthesis, melanin production, energy, and aids in the absorption of iron.
8. **Glass dishes, containers, and Tupperware.** Glass is primarily silica. It is healthier than plastic and other containers. Silica is great for strengthening bones, teeth, hair, skin, nails, joints, lungs, and all tissues and organs.
9. **Steamer baskets**. Stainless steel or bamboo steamer baskets enable wet heat cooking.
10. **Stone mortar and pestle**. A great way to grind fresh herbs and foods to add to meals or make medicine. Also a good source of the minerals silica, calcium, sodium, potassium, lithium, and others coming from the rock. Granite or marble are good choices.
11. **Sharp knives**. Dull knives can be more dangerous than sharp knives because they require more force and pressure to use.
12. **Real silver silverware**. Silver is antimicrobial. Eating with silver silverware can help to kill bad bacteria on poor quality food.
13. **Spring water**. Never use tap water when cooking; it is toxic. And spring water is full of minerals.
14. **Pit barbecuing.** Many traditional and indigenous cultures barbecue by wrapping food in banana leaves, flax leaves, maguey leaves, seaweed, or other methods and burying it underground in coals and dirt. Wrapped as such, these foods are almost steamed or en papillote cooked.
15. **Choose whole, fresh, wild, heirloom, organic, biodynamic-grown, permaculture-grown, home-grown, local, and/or wild-foraged foods as close to nature as possible**. Everything you eat should be medicinal. Every meal you eat should have fresh herbs/spices added to it. Every meal you eat should contain at least some raw foods.
16. **Do not wash most of your fruits and vegetables**. The skins of fruits and vegetables contain microbes that are necessary for their digestion and getting a diversity of microbes is important for a healthy gut. Also, food that is too sanitary may contribute to allergies and autoimmune conditions according to the "hygiene hypothesis".

# Growing Food

# Companion Planting & Growing Conditions Chart: 60+ Fruits, Vegetables, Herbs, & Spices

Collin Gow, C.N.C. (2021)

| Plant | Life Cycle | Companions | Enemies | PH | Sun | Growth | Water | Soil | Nativity & Hardy Zone |
|---|---|---|---|---|---|---|---|---|---|
| Aloe Vera | Perennial | Borage, scented geraniums, onion family, sow thistle, balm of Gilead, elderberry | | 7-8.5 | Full | 24-39in | Dry | Sandy or gravely soil w/ good drainage | Africa, Zones 8-11 |
| Andrographis | Annual | | | 6.8 | Full | 1-3ft, 160 days to mature | Dry | Well drained and slightly sandy | India, Sri Lanka, Asia, Zones 10-12 |
| Arugula | Annual | Dill, rosemary, lettuce | | 6-7 | Full | 1-2ft | Frequently | Fertile, well-drained | Mediterranean, Zones 3-11 |
| Astragalus | Perennial | | | 7 - 7.4 | Full/ part shade | 4ft | Regularly | Sandy, well drained | China, Korea, Mongolia, Temperate regions of Northern Hemisphere, Zones 5-9 |

| | | | | | | | | | |
|---|---|---|---|---|---|---|---|---|---|
| Bananas | Perennial | Chick peas, bush beans, soy beans, lima beans, mung beans, cowpeas, paw paw, sweet potatoes, pole beans, coffee beans, castor beans, comfrey, nasturtiums, papaya | | 5.5 - 6.5 | Full | 10ft - 23ft | Ample | Compost-rich, loamy, well-drained | Indomalaya, Australia, Papua New Guinea, Zones 9-10 |
| Basil | Annual, perennial in zones 10-11 | Apricot, asparagus, chives, cucumber, fennel, tomato, peppers, oregano, eggplant | Rue, rosemary, sage | 5.7 -7 | Full | 1-3ft | Moist | Fertile, well-drained | Central Africa to Southeast Asia, Zones 2-11 |
| Basil (Thai) | Annual | | | 6-7 | Full | 1-2ft, 80 days to mature | Moist | Rich, well draining | Southeast Asia |
| Black Eyed Peas | Annual | Cucumbers, luffa sponge, squash, pumpkins, melons, celery, strawberries, oregano, catnip, carrots, corn, radish | Onions, garlic, fennel | 5.5 - 6.5 | Full | 3ft | | Well drained loam, average fertility | Africa |

| | | | | | | | | | |
|---|---|---|---|---|---|---|---|---|---|
| Blueberries | Perennial | Oak, pine, rhododendron, potatoes, peppers, thyme, tomatoes, eggplant, okra, parsley, basil | | 4.3 - 5.5 | Full/ part shade | 6-12ft | Moist | Organic-matter rich, well-draining | North America |
| Beets | Biennial, infreq. perennial, often grown as an annual | Chives, garlic, leeks, onions, broccoli, Brussels sprouts, cabbage, cauliflower, lettuce, radish, spinach, asparagus, bush beans, peas, butter beans, mint, chard, savory, borage | Tomatoes, mustard, pole beans | 6-7.5 | Full sun and cool temp | 12-18in | | Sandy in spring, heavier in fall | Mediterranean |
| Borage | Annual | Tomatoes, squash, strawberry | | 6-7 | Full/ part shade | 3ft | | Well drained, moisture retentive, rich in organic matter | |

| | | | | | | | | | |
|---|---|---|---|---|---|---|---|---|---|
| Brassicas | | Chamomile, dill, mint, rosemary, sage, lettuce, borage, beets, carrots, oregano, spinach, buckwheat, chives, cucumber | Tomatoes, peppers, potatoes, eggplant, corn, asparagus, pumpkins, grapes, strawberries, radishes, watermel., mustards, pole beans | 6-7 | | | | Fertile with extra calcium and nitrogen | |
| Butcher's Broom | Perennial | | | Any, 6.1 - 7.8 | Part shade to full shade | 1-3ft | Moist best, but adaptable | Any | Eurasia, North Africa, Zones 7-9 |
| Carrots | Biennial or annual | Leeks, radish, onions, parsley, lettuce, tomato, rosemary, sage | Dill, celery | | | 12in | | No heavy or stony soils. Ideally friable, well-drained. | |
| Catnip | Perennial | Potatoes, eggplant, beets, pumpkin, squash, hyssop, collards, parsley, tomatoes, Brassicas, okra | | 6.1 - 7.8 | Sun/ part shade | 1-4ft | Dryish | Moderately rich loam or sandy with good drainage | Southern and Eastern Europe, Middle East, Central Asia, Parts of China |

| | | | | | | | | | |
|---|---|---|---|---|---|---|---|---|---|
| Celery | Biennial | Bush beans, broccoli, cauliflower, leeks, onion, cabbage family, tomato, cucumber, spinach, marjoram, cosmos, daisies, marigolds, nasturtiums, snapdragons | Carrots, corn, potatoes, parsley, parsnips, turnips | 5.8 - 6.8 | Does not like heat. 60-70 deg. ideal | 18-24in | Needs constant watering | Rich, fertile, with plenty of organic matter | |
| Chamomile | Roman is perennial, German is annual | Plant throughout garden | | | | 8-24in | | Well-drained, sandy (German) | |
| Chives | Perennial | Carrots, tomato, marigold, basil, strawberry, parsnip | Beans, cucumber, peas | 6-7 | Full sun | 8in -2ft clumps | Moist, water frequently | Loamy, sandy | Temperate areas of Europe, Asia, and North America |
| Cilantro | Annual | Beans, peas, spinach, tomato, potatoes, asparagus, chervil, basil, mint, yarrow, tansy, jalapeno peppers, onion, lettuce, chervil, cruciferous, carrots, anise, corn | Fennel | 6.1 - 7.2 | Full sun/ part shade | 1-2ft branching | Water every 2-4 days | Rich, well draining | Southern Europe, Northern Africa, Southwestern Asia |

| | | | | | | | | | |
|---|---|---|---|---|---|---|---|---|---|
| Citrus | Perennial | Lemon balm, dill, marigolds, garlic, dandelion, thyme | | | | | | | |
| Cucumber | Annual | Beans, chamomile, corn, English pea, leek, lettuce, onion, radish, sunflower, celery, marigold, dill, nasturtium | Chives, aromatic herbs, Irish potato | | | 1-7ft | | | |
| Dill | Biennial | Cabbage, lettuce, onion, kale, rosemary | Carrots, cucumber, tomato, cilantro | 5.1 - 6.5 | Full/ part sun | 2-3ft upright | Let soil go dry betwe en wateri ngs | Loose, not too fertile soil | Eurasia |

| | | | | | | | | | |
|---|---|---|---|---|---|---|---|---|---|
| Echinacea | Perennial | Lemon balm, catmint, gentian, salvia (Mealy Blue Sage), lavender, butterfly weed, goat's beard, beard tongue, bee balm, aloe, butterfly milkweed, false sunflower, hoary skullcap, purple poppy mallow, black-eyed Susan, | | 5.6-7 | Full/ part sun | 3-5ft | Dryish | Adaptable | Eastern and Central North America |
| Fennel | Perennial | Most plants dislike it | Beans, peppers, tomatoes, cilantro, caraway, dill, kohlrabi, tomatoes | 6.1-8 | Full sun | 1.5-2ft | Regular watering | Well drained, deep, moderately fertile | |
| Garlic | Biennial | Beets, cabbage, tomatoes, onions, raspberries, strawberries, apple, apricot, cherry, mulberry, rosemary, roses | Beans, peas | 6-7 | Full sun | 2ft upright | Dry | Sandy loam loose well draining | Central Asia, Northeastern Iran |

| | | | | | | | | | |
|---|---|---|---|---|---|---|---|---|---|
| Ginger | Perennial | Chili peppers, cilantro, lemongrass, red clover, kaffir lime, beans, peas, galangal, turmeric, hibiscus, palms, orchids | | 5-7 | | 2-4ft upright | Moist | | |
| Jalapeno | Grown as annual but perennial in zones 9-11 | | | 6-6.8 | Full sun | 2-4ft | Every other day | Nutrient rich, good drainage | Mexico |
| Kale | Biennial | Dill, rosemary, garlic, onions, artichokes, beets, celery, cucumbers, lettuce, onion, peas, potatoes, radishes, spinach, spinach, basil, chamomile, dill, mint, sage, rosemary, thyme, catnip | Strawberry, tomato | 6-7 | Full sun | 2-3ft | | Loamy | |

| | | | | | | | | | |
|---|---|---|---|---|---|---|---|---|---|
| Lavender | Perennial | All plants benefit from it. Chamomile, lettuce, Brassicas, onions, tomatoes, oregano, thyme, marjoram, sage, rosemary, basil, lemon balm, squash, olive, fruit trees | Not compatible with plants that need lots of water or lots of shade | 6.5 - 7.5 | | 20-24in | | | |
| Lemon Balm | Perennial | Basil, tomatoes, lettuce, oregano, chives, okra, cabbage, carrots, radishes, squashes, berries, fruit trees, cantaloupe, watermelon, sage, thyme, parsley, marjoram | Sprinkle throughout garden | 5.8 -7 | Full/ part sun | 2ft | Moist, yet well draining, is not drought resistant | Loose loam/sandy loam | South-central Europe, Mediterranean Basin, Iran, Central Asia, and now Naturalized in the Americas |
| Lettuce | Annual | Carrots, chard, cucumber, dill, peas, radish, strawberry, beans, beets, marigold | Pole beans, tomatoes, parsley | 6-7 | Full/ part sun, does not like too much heat | 1ft | | Well drained, cool, loose soil | |

| | | | | | | | | | |
|---|---|---|---|---|---|---|---|---|---|
| Leeks | Biennial | Carrots, celery, cucumber, onion, lettuce | Bush beans, pole beans, peas | | | 2-3ft | | | |
| Licorice | Tropical Perennial in zones 9-11 | Marigold, marjoram, rosemary, lettuce, | Onion, leek, garlic, cruciferous | 6-8 | Full/ part sun | 5ft, 2-4 years to mature | Moist | Light, loamy, well drained | Mediterra nean, Southern and Central Russia, Asia Minor, Iran |
| Marigold (Calendula) | Annual | Basil, cucumber, eggplant, gourd, tomatoes, kale, potatoes, squash, melons, lettuce, asparagus, onion, chard, radish, carrots, tomatoes, thyme, parsley, plant throughout garden | Beans, cabbage | | | 6in-2ft | | | |
| Mint | Perennial | Cabbage, pea, tomato | Cucumber | | | 18-36in | | | |
| Milk Thistle | Biennial | | | 6.1 - 6.5 | | 12-79in | | | Southern Europe, Asia |

| | | | | | | | | | |
|---|---|---|---|---|---|---|---|---|---|
| Nettles (Stinging) | Perennial | Tomatoes, cruciferous, herbs, vegetables, Peppermint, tomatoes, broccoli, lemon balm, chamomile, oregano, mint, sage | | 5.5 - 7.5 | Full/ part sun | 3-6ft | Moist | Slightly damp, rich in nitrogen, rich, well drained loam, edges of streams or nutrient dense pastures | Europe, Temperate Asia and North Africa |
| Okinawa Spinach | | Brassicas, eggplant, leeks, lettuce, peas, radish, strawberry | Potatoes | | Full | 2ft | | | |
| Okra | Tropical Perennial, annual in temperate climates | Peppers, tomatoes, beans, radishes, lettuce, catnip, basil, peas, eggplant, marigolds | | | | 3-6ft | | | |
| Onion | Biennial | Beets, broccoli, cabbage, carrots, cauliflower, celery, chamomile, chard, chives, cucumber, dill, leeks, lettuce, summer savory, strawberry, garlic | Beans, English peas, sage | | | 15-36in | | | |

| | | | | | | | | | |
|---|---|---|---|---|---|---|---|---|---|
| Oregano | | Pumpkins, tomatoes, peppers, cabbage, grapes | Cucumber | 6.5 -7 | | 1-2ft | | | Mediterranean, Western Asia, Naturalized in Mexico and U.S. |
| Oregano (Cuban) | Perennial | | | 7 | Full/ part sun | 2ft | Let dry out completely between waterings | Fast draining, nutrient rich, gritty soil | |
| Parsley | Biennial | Tomatoes, asparagus, carrots, chives, corn, onion, peppers, peas, beans, chives, rosemary, roses, celery, kale, spinach, strawberries, apple | Lettuce, some alliums, mint | 5.5 - 6.7 | Full/ part sun | 1-1.5ft | Adaptable | Nutrient rich, well draining | Central and Eastern Mediterranean, Naturalized in Europe |
| Purslane | | carrots, cabbage, beets, radishes, turnips, lettuce, basil, corn | | | | 4-8in | | | |

| | | | | | | | | | |
|---|---|---|---|---|---|---|---|---|---|
| Hot Peppers | Perennial in hot zones, annual in cooler zones | Basil, okra, carrots, cucumber, coriander, onion, spinach, tomato | Fennel, beans | 6-6.8 | | 1.5-2ft | | | |
| Peppermint | Perennial in zones 3-11 | Mint family plants, alliums, Brassicas, cabbage, peas, tomatoes | | | | 1-3ft | | | |
| Potato (Irish) | Perennial grown as an annual | Beans, broccoli, cabbage, cauliflower, corn, eggplant, horseradish, marigolds, celery nasturtiums, thyme, garlic, horseradish, onions, peas, spinach, radish, basil | Cucumber, melon, pumpkin, squash, sunflower, turnip, tomato | 4.8 - 5.5 | Full | 3-4ft | Every 2 days | Well drained, loose | Americas |
| Prickly pear | Perennial | Agave, echinacea | | | | 10-15ft | | | Americas |
| Pumpkins | | Melons, squash, garlic, onion, thyme, sage, mint, lavender, dill, oregano, marigold, nasturtiums, corn, beans | Potato | | | 1-3ft | | | |

| | | | | | | | | | |
|---|---|---|---|---|---|---|---|---|---|
| Radish | Annual or biennial | Carrots, cucumber, English pea, lettuce, Nasturtium | | | | 6in-18in | | | |
| Rosemary | Perennial in zones 7-10 | Beans, kale, cabbage, sage, thyme, broccoli, | Basil, potatoes, pumpkins | 6-7 | Full | 3-4ft | Dry | Loamy, sandy, or rock | Mediterra nean |
| Squash | Annual | Borage, corn, marigold, nasturtium, beans, peas, dill, strawberry, sunflower | Irish potato | | | | | | |
| Sweet potatoes | Annual in most zones, perennial in zones 9-11 | Dill, parsnips, beets, potatoes, bush beans | | 5.5 - 6.5 | | 20ft spread | | | |
| Sage | Perennial in zones 5-8, annual in zones 9 and further south | Strawberries, tomatoes, carrots, cabbage, oregano, beans, peas, rosemary, roses | Cucumber | 6-6.5 | Full sun, but does not like heat | 2-3ft | Dry | Rich, well draining, light or heavy | Mediterra nean |
| Spider plant | Perennial in 9-11, annual in other zones | | Potatoes, onions, carrots, garlic, turnips | | | 12-15in | | | |

| | | | | | | | | | |
|---|---|---|---|---|---|---|---|---|---|
| Strawberry | Short term perennial | Borage, lettuce, onion, sage, spinach, thyme, bush beans, chives, squash, caraway, sage | Broccoli, cabbage, cauliflower, eggplant, tomato, potato, peppers | 5.5 - 6.9 | | 6-8in | | | |
| Tomato | Perennial, yet grown as annuals | Asparagus, basil, borage, carrots, celery, chives, cucumber, garlic, onion marigold, mint, nasturtium, onion, parsley, sage, thyme, lettuce, spinach | Broccoli, cabbage, cauliflower, corn, dill, fennel, potato, kohlrabi, lettuce, beets, cruciferous, peas, rosemary | 5.6 -7 | Full | 3-4ft | | | |
| Turmeric | Perennial | Eggplant, peppers, tomatoes, ginger, corn, chili, pigeon pea | | | | 3.3ft | | | |
| Turnip | Biennial | English pea | Potato, mustard | | | 12-18in | | | |
| Thyme | Perennial in zones 5-9 | Gets along with most plants, eggplant, potato, strawberry, tomato, broccoli, cauliflower | Oregano, onion, garlic, marjoram, turnip | 5.8 - 7.5 | Full/ part sun | 6-15in | Moist | Loamy, sandy, well drained, rich in organic matter | Temperate regions of Europe, North Africa, and Asia |

| | | | | | | | | | |
|---|---|---|---|---|---|---|---|---|---|
| Watercress | Perennial | Chives, peppermint, wintergreen,s pearmint | | | | 2-24in | | | |
| Wormwood | Annual | As a border, keeps animals out, carrots, onions, leek, sage, rosemary, Brassicas | Anise, beans, caraway, fennel, peas, sage | An y | Full/ part sun | 1-3ft, Fast growing | Dry, yet good to mulch | Not rich soil, sandy and loamy soils, well drained | Temperat e Asia |

# Natural Ways to Deter Pests and Animals From Your Garden

Collin Gow, C.N.C.

3/17/2021

| Pests & Animals | Deterrents |
|---|---|
| Rabbits | Echinacea, nasturtiums, hair clippings, alyssum, marigolds, garlic, peppers, dish soap, wind chime or cans on a string, daffodil, sage, asparagus, yarrow, black-eyed Susan, rosemary, onions, lemon balm, lavender, English ivy, thyme, keep garden open so nowhere to hide, let cats or dogs roam around the property, 1/2"X1/2" wire mesh 3' high and 3' deep |
| Squirrels | Daffodils, crown imperials, garlic, onions, scallions, fritilaries, galanthus, hyacinth, lily of the valley, geraniums, squirrel baffle |
| Aphids, Whiteflies, Cabbage Worms, Mealybugs, Mosquitoes, Nematodes, Moths, Cockroaches, Termites, Scale, Snails, Gnats | Neem oil |
| Mice | Lavender, catnip, mint |
| Raccoons | Squash, cucumber, oriental poppies, chili pepper |
| Deer | Sage, dill, oregano |
| Grasshoppers, Mosquitoes, Flies | Frogs |
| Snakes | Andrographis |
| Ants | Cayenne, baking soda, coffee grounds, dish soap, chickens, fragrant herbs, mint, lemon, cinnamon, marigolds, tansy, garlic, rosemary, lavender, thyme, sage, lemongrass, catnip, yarrow |
| Birds | Cayenne pepper spray, shiny metallic objects in the wind such as a pinwheel, paint rocks as fake berries, fake snakes, scarecrow, garlic oil spray, lots of coconut trees for miles as they do not nest in them, noises, fake owls and hawks with sound chips in them that produce predator sounds, planting sunflowers on the opposite side of your fruit trees to feed the birds, add a bird feeder away from trees to attract birds to feeder instead of berries, bird netting. Birds may eat unwanted insects however. |
| All Pests (but can kill all beneficial insects also) | Diatomaceous earth |

# Pharmaceutical Drugs

# Nutrients Depleted
# By Pharmaceutical Drugs

Collin Gow, C.N.C. (2021)

| | |
|---|---|
| Acid blockers/PPIs (Omeprazole, Pantoprazole) | All nutrients |
| Aluminum antacids (Gaviscon, Maalox, Mylanta) | Vitamin A, folic acid, vitamin D, calcium, chromium, iron, magnesium, phosphorus, zinc |
| Antibiotics (Amoxicillin, Doxycycline) | B-vitamins, calcium, magnesium, iron, vitamin K, zinc, healthy bacteria |
| Antidepressants - MAO inhibitors (Isocarboxazid, Phenelzine) | Vitamin B6 |
| Antidepressants - SSRIs (Fluoxetine, Citalopram, Sertraline) | Iodine, melatonin |
| Antidepressants - Tricyclics (Amitriptyline) | CoQ10, vitamin B2 |
| Anxiety medications - Benzodiazepines (Lorazepam, Diazepam) | Melatonin |
| Autoimmune/Anti-inflammatory medications - Corticosteroids (Prednisone) | Vitamins A, C, D, K, B6, B2, folic acid, calcium, magnesium, selenium, potassium, zinc |
| Blood pressure medications - ACE inhibitors (Lisinopril) | Sodium, zinc, magnesium, potassium, calcium |
| Blood pressure medications - Angiotensin II receptor blockers (sartans, eg. Losartan) | Magnesium, phosphorus, potassium, sodium, zinc, CoQ10 |
| Blood pressure medications - Beta-blockers (Carvedilol, Metoprolol) | CoQ10, melatonin |
| Blood pressure medications - Calcium channel blockers (Amlodipine) | Potassium, vitamin D, calcium, possibly CoQ10 |
| Blood pressure medications (Clonidine, Methyldopa) | CoQ10 |
| Breathing medications - synthetic glucocorticoids (Budesonide) | Folic acid, most minerals, iodine |
| Cholesterol medications - Bile acid sequestrants (Cholestyramine) | beta-carotene, folic acid, vitamin A, B12, vitamins D, E, and K, iron |
| Cholesterol medications - Fibrates (Fenofibrate) | Most minerals, B-vitamins |
| Cholesterol medications - Statins (Atorvastatin, Rosuvastatin) | CoQ10, possibly vitamin D |
| Diabetes medications (Glyburide) | CoQ10, B12, folic acid, sodium |
| Diabetes medications (Metformin) | CoQ10, B6, B12, folic acid |
| Diuretics | B-vitamins, vitamin C, zinc, calcium, magnesium, potassium |
| Gout medications (Colchicine) | Vitamin A, B12, potassium, calcium |
| Laxatives - Bisacodyl (Dulcolax) | Potassium, other minerals |
| Laxatives - Magnesium Hydroxide (Milk of Magnesia) | Folic acid, vitamin D, calcium, iron, phosphorus, zinc |
| Laxatives - Mineral oil | Vitamin A, calcium, vitamin D, vitamin E, many other nutrients |
| NSAIDs (Ibuprofen, Naproxen, Ketoprofen, Meloxicam) | vitamin C, folic acid, iron |
| Oral contraceptives, estrogen hormone replacement therapy | Healthy flora, magnesium, zinc, most minerals, B-vitamins, vitamin C |
| Pain medications (Hydrocodone plus Acetaminophen) | Glutathione, selenium |
| Salicylates (Aspirin, Percodan, Fiorinal) | Vitamin C, calcium, iron, folic acid, pantethine, protein |
| Seizure medications - Sodium channel blockers (Phenytoin) | Biotin, folic acid, B1, B12, vitamins D, and K, calcium, phosphorus, carnitine |
| Thyroid medications (Levothyroxine, Synthroid, Armour) | Iron, calcium |

# Articles

# Medical Astrology: Cell Salts and Herbs For Each Sign (Constellation) of the Zodiac

Collin Gow, C.N.C.

3/13/2022

Each sign (constellation) of the zodiac corresponds to a certain region and function of the body and certain body parts, which rely on particular cell salts. It is considered by some, that the sign in which your sun is located in your natal chart, is the most important sign, linking your most needed cell salt in medical astrology. However, some ancient eastern astrologers believed that the rising sign was the most important sign, therefore the cell salt associated with one's rising sign is important as well. I would consider one's moon sign and other factors in the natal chart too. Either way, you do need more than 1 cell salt (which usually consists of **two minerals, but not always**) for your overall health. There are **12 cell salts** that are considered **essential** within Homeopathy. However, you may find yourself craving foods that are high in the cell salts associated with your strongest signs and elemental energies within your natal chart. Each sign of the the **12 signs in the Zodiac** requires more of its associated cell salt because the body part/chakra and body function associated with a particular sign, which requires that cell salt to function, is more active, therefore that cell salt is used up more rapidly. Whether you "believe" in astrology or not, I find medical astrology to be very accurate, just as I find blood type diets and some other ways of personalizing nutrition to be accurate. You decide for yourself. Nevertheless, it's important to personalize your nutrition to your own unique biochemical individuality. Medical astrology is one way to do that.

**The signs and their cell salts are as follows:**

## Cell Salts

**Aries** is ruled by the head/brain, cerebrum, spinal chord, sensory nerves, face, eyes, and is associated with the cell salt Kali Phos or potassium phosphate.

**Taurus** is ruled by the neck/throat, ears, larynx, tonsils, liver, gallbladder, cerebellum and is associated with Nat Sulph or sodium sulfate.

**Gemini** is ruled by the chest, arms, shoulders, lungs, pleura, bronchial tubes, fibers, tissues, hands and is associated with Kali mur or potassium chloride.

**Cancer** is ruled by the stomach, breasts, spleen, upper liver, elastic tissue and is associated with calcarea fluorica or calcium fluoride.

**Leo** is ruled by the heart, motor nerves, back and side near the heart, and is associated with Mag phos or magnesium phosphate.

**Virgo** is ruled by the bowels, solar plexus, and lower liver and is associated with Kali sulph or potassium sulfate.

**Libra** is ruled by the kidneys, bladder, appendix, and skin and is associated with Nat phos or sodium phosphate.

**Scorpio** is ruled by the genitals/loins and vascular coatings and casts, and is associated with Calcarea sulphate or calcium sulfate.

**Sagittarius** is ruled by the hips and thighs, sciatic nerves, and is associated with Silica.

**Capricorn** is ruled by the bones, teeth, hair, knees, sacrum and is associated with Calcarea phosphate or calcium phosphate.

**Aquarius** is ruled by the lower legs, ankles, shins, calfs, and white blood cells and the circulatory system and is associate with Nat mur or sodium chloride or table salt.

**Pisces** is ruled by the feet, arterial blood, and red blood cells and is associated with Ferrum phos or iron phosphate.

**Each constellation and planet is associated with an herb as well:**

## Herbs

**Aries:** Hops, nettles, gentian, cayenne, butcher's broom, garlic, honeysuckle, blessed thistle.

**Taurus:** Sage, Thyme, Plantain, Coltsfoot, Tansy, Silverweed, Goldenrod, Bearberry.

**Gemini:** Scullcap, Lily of the Valley, Flaxseed, Parsley, Meadowsweet, Caraway, Lavender.

**Cancer:** Water Lily, Chickweed, Honeysuckle, Dog's Tooth, Lettuce.

**Leo:** Eyebright, St. John's Wort, Mistletoe, Marigold, Wake Robin, Walnuts.

**Virgo:** Scullcap, Fennel, Licorice, Dill, Mandrake, Pellitory of the Wall, Endive.

**Libra:** Pennyroyal, Violet, Thyme, Feverfew, Catmint, Silverweed, Archangel, Bearberry, Burdock.

**Scorpio:** Horehound, Blessed Thislte, Horse Radish, Toad Flax, Leek, Wormwood, Sarsaparilla, Blackberry Leaves.

**Sagittarius:** Agrimony, Red Clover, Burdock, Podophyllum, May Apple, Chicory, Dandelion, Oak.

**Capricorn:** Comfrey, Horsetail, Shavegrass, Knot Grass, Slippery Elm, Thuja, Shepherd's Purse, Wintergreen, Fumitory, Thyme.

**Aquarius:** Valerian, Lady's Slipper, Snakeroot, Southernwood.

**Pisces:** Seaweeds such as kelp, dulse, bladderwrack, Irish moss, etc.

# Protocols

# Allergies

Collin Gow, C.N.C.

1/8/2022

**Allergies** occur when the body overreacts to antigens (proteins) from normally harmless substances.[1] Common allergens include: **pollen, dust mites, pets, farm animals, venom in insect stings/bites, foods, medications**, contact "allergens" such as **metals** or **fragrance** ingredients, **herbicides, pesticides, and mold**.[1,2] Typical symptoms include runny nose, coughing, sneezing, itching, breathing problems, watery eyes, rash, swollen mucus membranes, and gastrointestinal problems. Other symptoms such as swelling of the lips or tongue, nausea, vomiting, abdominal cramps, and syncope can occur as well. Common food allergens include **dairy, egg whites, shellfish, peanuts, tree nuts, soy, wheat, and fish**. Pick 3 or 4 of the following.

### "Herbal" Supplements/Polyphenols

**Amla** inhibited histidine decarboxylase, an enzyme that catalyzes the synthesis of histamine, by as much as 90% in one study.[3] It is also a good source of vitamin C. **Butterbur** was studied against cetirizine (the antihistamine in Zyrtec) in 2002 and shown to be equally as effective.[4] ***Tinospora cordifolia*** is an Ayurvedic, adaptogenic, immunomodulating herb that has traditionally been used to increase immune defenses against malaria, infection, and liver toxicity, yet it also reduces the immune response to allergies, inflammation, arthritis, and fever. It reduces eosinophils, neutrophils, and goblet cells, cells involved in allergies, inflammation, and mucus, respectively. It also reduces nasal obstruction, runny nose, and itchy nose.[5-9] **Boswellia** may be beneficial for food allergies that are triggering colitis. **Licorice** raises cortisol which may help to stabilize the cell membrane of lysosomes (ruptured lysosomes cause the inflammation that occurs in an allergic response). **Quercetin** and **pycnogenol** may stabilize the cell membranes of mast cells (mast cells release histamine in response to antigens). **Resveratrol** inhibits the activation of eosinophils. **Elderberry flowers** contain ursolic acid, which may inhibit mast cell degranulation and histamine release.

### Aminos

**Histidine** may increase the production of T-suppressor cells. More T-suppressor cells are associated with less allergies. **Methionine** may inhibit the secretion of excess histamine.

### Vitamins

**Vitamin B6** is a cofactor for histaminase, an enzyme which breaks down histamine. Pick the P-5-P, coenzymated form of B6. **Vitamin D3** may be helpful for allergies, especially in children and adolescents. **Vitamin C** may reduce histamine release. Amla is the best choice for a vitamin C source for allergies.

### Minerals

**Zinc** may inhibit histamine release from mast cells and basophils and the activity of series 4 leukotrienes that activate the inflammation involved in an allergic response. Take no more than 15mg at a time, as excess can cause nausea. **MSM** and **iodine** are good also. There are anecdotal reports that iodine has been helpful for fruit sensitivities/allergies.

### EFAs

**Omega 3·6·9s** may help to reduce the inflammation in allergies and soothe the mucus membranes.

### Probiotics/Prebiotics

Probiotics, especially **soil-based organisms** (soil-based organisms are capable of shifting Th2 immunity to Th1 immunity, a less hyperallergic side of immunity). However, one should not take these everyday, long-term. They are to be used temporarily and/or cycled.

### Enzymes

**Pancreatin** may help to digest antigens in foods, making them less likely to react with your immune system.

### Foods

Allspice, oysters, pumpkin seeds, vitamin D fortified mushrooms, apples, onions, berries, cabbage, buckwheat, seaweeds, fatty fish, bee pollen, and raw honey are good. Hot peppers and citrus fruits are high in vitamin C, but many people are sensitive to them. Limit refined and processed foods.

References:

1. InformedHealth.org [Internet]. Cologne, Germany: Institute for Quality and Efficiency in Health Care (IQWiG); 2006-. Allergies: Overview. [Updated 2020 Apr 23]. Available from: https://www.ncbi.nlm.nih.gov/books/NBK447112/
2. Hoppin, Jane A et al. "Pesticides are Associated with Allergic and Non-Allergic Wheeze among Male Farmers." *Environmental health perspectives* vol. 125,4 (2017): 535-543. doi:10.1289/EHP315
3. Nitta, Yoko et al. "Novel inhibitors for histidine decarboxylase from plant components." (2017).
4. Schapowal, Andreas. (2002). Randomized controlled trial of butterbur and cetirizine for treating seasonal allergic rhinitis. BMJ (Clinical research ed.). 324. 144-6. 10.1136/bmj.324.7330.144.
5. Thawani VR, Badar VA, Gharpure KJ, Wakode PT, Hingorani LL. Short term effect of Tinospora cordifolia in allergic rhinitis. The Antiseptic. 2006 April;103(4&P):229-32.
6. Sharma U, Bala M, Kumar N, Singh B, Munshi RK, Bhalerao S. Immunomodulatory active compounds from Tinospora cordifolia. J Ethnopharmacol. 2012 Jun 14;141(3):918-26. Epub 2012 Mar 26.
7. Upadhyay AK, Kumar K, Kumar A, Mishra HS. Tinospora cordifolia (Willd.) Hook. f. and Thoms. (Guduchi) – validation of the Ayurvedic pharmacology through experimental and clinical studies. Int J Ayurveda Res. 2010 Apr-Jun;1(2):112–121.
8. Wadood N, Wadood A, Shah SA. Effect of Tinospora cordifolia on blood glucose and total lipid levels of normal and alloxan-diabetic rabbits. Planta Medica. 1992;58:31-136.
9. Sharma V, Pandey D. Protective Role of Tinospora cordifolia against lead-induced hepatotoxicity. Toxicol Int. 2010 Jan;17(1):12-7.

# Bones and Teeth

Collin Gow, C.N.C.
2/20/2022

Bones and teeth are both hard, calcium rich tissues. Though bones are higher in collagen and have a better ability to heal on their own than teeth, some of the same natural compounds may be useful for both. Furthermore, osteoporosis and periodontal disease have common risk factors,[1] similar metabolic disturbances may affect both, and lower bone mineral density has been associated with cavities.[2] Osteoporosis is a state of low bone mineral density, loss of bone mass, and deterioration of the bones. 50% of white, postmenopausal women and 20% of white men will experience a fracture related to osteoporosis.[3] Biphosphonates are the most commonly prescribed drugs for osteoporosis. There are two key cells involved in bone health—osteoclasts and osteoblasts. **Osteoclasts break down bone (bone resorption). Osteoblasts build bone**. Cavities (dental caries) are a chronic, infectious, transmissible disease caused primarily by the bacteria Streptococcus mutans, which produces acid that demineralizes the teeth.[4] **Cavities are the most common ailment in the United States affecting 2.3 billion people.**[5,6] Conventional treatments consist of oral hygeine (brushing and flossing), topical fluoride gels, sealants, and fillings. However, natural medicines and diet and lifestyle changes are preferred by some for bone health and teeth health. Here is a review of some of those stand-outs and their effects.

**Supplements:**
A bone building product containing algae-sourced **calcium,** along with **silica, magnesium, vitamin D3, vitamin K2 (menaquinone-7), and boron** may be helpful for bones and teeth. Calcium, silica, magnesium, and boron mineralize bones and teeth, making them stronger. Magnesium helps to keep calcium in solution so it doesn't crystallize in soft tissue and contribute to plaque formation in the arteries instead of building bone. Magnesium also assists in vitamin D3 absorption. Vitamin D3 aids in the absorption of calcium from the stomach into the blood, inhibits osteoclasts, and activates osteoblasts. Vitamin K2 gets the calcium from the blood into the bones and teeth. K2 also increases matrix GLA protein, which makes calcified plaque in the arteries more pliable. It is important to have flexible arteries. Silica concentrates in bones and is involved in the synthesis of collagen; it creates a mesh matrix that holds collagen together. Silica is like the mortar of the body. Collagen is like the bricks. This silica/collagen matrix is an important component of bone tissue. Silica reduces tooth decay and speeds the healing of fractures by facilitating the incorporation and retention of calcium in teeth and bones. There is also some conjecture that silica can transmute into calcium in the body. Boron concentrates in the parathyroid glands, affects cell membrane transport of calcium, and is essential to convert vitamin D2 (inactive vitamin D) to vitamin D3 (active vitamin D). **The parathyroid glands regulate the level of calcium in your blood and bones and the level of phosphorous in serum**. **Potassium** is great too. It reduces bone resorption. Getting potassium from foods is better than potassium from supplements. **Morphogenic bone protein (milk-based protein)** may help to build bone as well, however, I generally recommend consuming organic soy or organic fermented soy instead. **Strontium** makes bones hard, but brittle, like glass, so I don't recommend supplementing with extra strontium beyond what naturally may occur in an algae-sourced calcium product. Many people think that calcium is bad for you. In isolation, it may be, but when combined with the other necessary nutrients listed above that it needs to work properly, it is beneficial. It aids the contraction of muscles and strengthens bones and teeth. Your body can't make it to any large degree, so it is considered an essential mineral that is required in relatively high amounts compared to other minerals. **Vitamin A** deficiency can cause impaired tooth formation and enamel hypoplasia (underdeveloped enamel).[7]

Consider taking your **probiotics once a week, not every day**. While some studies show that *Lactobacilli* can be anti-cariogenic, other studies show that *Lactobacilli* are cariogenic.[8] Premature grey hair has been linked to a higher rate of osteoporosis. **Copper** could be the link here, as it may be helpful for grey hair and also for collagen synthesis, which may strengthen bones. **Zinc** deficiency can impair bone growth. Take no more than 25mg per pill, any higher per pill may cause nausea in some people.

**Anti-Streptococcus mutans activity: cacao bean husk** (*in vitro and in vivo*),[9] alcohol **extract of eucalyptus twigs** and alcohol extract of **mango twigs**,[10] **Cinnamon oil, lemongrass oil, and cedarwood oil** (*in vitro*),[11] **Coriander essential oil** (anti-biofilm), Whitebrush essential oil (anti-biofilm), alecrim pimenta essential oil (anti-biofilm), alecrim do campo essential oil (anti-biofilm),[12] alcohol **extract of holy basil** (*in vitro*), **asparagus extract** (*in vitro*), **rosemary essential oil** (anti-biofilm) (*in vivo*).[6]

**Foods:** Eat a more **alkaline diet** consisting of high amounts of fruits and vegetables. Excessive amounts of acidic foods, especially without supplementing alkaline minerals, rob your bones and teeth of calcium. Consume **rosemary** and **asparagus**. Consume **cranberries**, though they are slightly acidic, they are also anti-cariogenic.[13] Eat organic, fermented or non-fermented **soy** 3 times per week. Isoflavones in soy have been well-established to diminish bone resorption and aid in the formation of bones.[14] **Natto** (fermented soy) has been associated with reduced tooth loss.[15] Don't eat too many crunchy, processed foods that are high in refined sugar or sucrose. Eat **liver** once a week for vitamin A.

**Lifestyle:** Weight bearing **exercise** helps to strengthen bones. Take one of the doses of your bone support supplement before bed. Most bone is lost while sleeping. For oral health, consider Swiss **biological dentistry**, **floss with ozonated oil**, use a **natural toothpaste** with xylitol and minerals, use a **natural mouthwash**, and try **oil pulling**. The **most important time to brush your teeth is before bed** because less saliva is produced while sleeping. Saliva helps control bad bacteria. **Opt out of root canals** so you're not leaving dead teeth in your mouth. Root canal endotoxins have been linked to periodontitis, an increased risk of depression, and coronary heart disease.[16,17] **Do not smoke cigarettes**. They contain cadmium. Cadmium interferes with bone formation. Fruit consumption may reduce cadmium levels in the body.[18]


1. Kaye EK. Bone health and oral health. J Am Dent Assoc. 2007 May;138(5):616-9. doi: 10.14219/jada.archive.2007.0232. PMID: 17473039.
2. Rezazadeh F, Emad S, Emad M. Relationship between Bone Mineral Density and Oral Health Status among Iranian Women. Int J Prev Med. 2019 Sep 5;10:149. doi: 10.4103/ijpvm.IJPVM_314_18. PMID: 31579164; PMCID: PMC6767921.
3. Porter JL, Varacallo M. Osteoporosis. [Updated 2021 Jul 18]. In: StatPearls [Internet]. Treasure Island (FL): StatPearls Publishing; 2022 Jan-. Available from: https://www.ncbi.nlm.nih.gov/books/NBK441901/
4. Rathee M, Sapra A. Dental Caries. [Updated 2021 Oct 6]. In: StatPearls [Internet]. Treasure Island (FL): StatPearls Publishing; 2022 Jan-. Available from: https://www.ncbi.nlm.nih.gov/books/NBK551699/
5. Heng C. Tooth Decay Is the Most Prevalent Disease. Fed Pract. 2016 Oct;33(10):31-33. PMID: 30766141; PMCID: PMC6373711.
6. Kumar M, Prakash S, Radha, Kumari N, Pundir A, Punia S, Saurabh V, Choudhary P, Changan S, Dhumal S, Pradhan PC, Alajil O, Singh S, Sharma N, Ilakiya T, Singh S, Mekhemar M.

Beneficial Role of Antioxidant Secondary Metabolites from Medicinal Plants in Maintaining Oral Health. Antioxidants (Basel). 2021 Jun 30;10(7):1061. doi: 10.3390/antiox10071061. PMID: 34209152; PMCID: PMC8300643.
7. Tungare S, Paranjpe AG. Diet and Nutrition To Prevent Dental Problems. [Updated 2021 Aug 11]. In: StatPearls [Internet]. Treasure Island (FL): StatPearls Publishing; 2022 Jan-. Available from: https://www.ncbi.nlm.nih.gov/books/NBK534248/
8. Badet C, Thebaud NB. Ecology of lactobacilli in the oral cavity: a review of literature. Open Microbiol J. 2008;2:38-48. doi: 10.2174/1874285800802010038. Epub 2008 Apr 29. PMID: 19088910; PMCID: PMC2593047.
9. Palombo EA. Traditional Medicinal Plant Extracts and Natural Products with Activity against Oral Bacteria: Potential Application in the Prevention and Treatment of Oral Diseases. Evid Based Complement Alternat Med. 2011;2011:680354. doi: 10.1093/ecam/nep067. Epub 2011 Jan 12. PMID: 19596745; PMCID: PMC3145422.
10. Banavar Ravi S, Nirupad S, Chippagiri P, Pandurangappa R. Antibacterial Effects of Natural Herbal Extracts on Streptococcus mutans: Can They Be Potential Additives in Dentifrices? Int J Dent. 2017;2017:4921614. doi: 10.1155/2017/4921614. Epub 2017 Oct 19. PMID: 29201054; PMCID: PMC5671721.
11. Chaudhari LK, Jawale BA, Sharma S, Sharma H, Kumar CD, Kulkarni PA. Antimicrobial activity of commercially available essential oils against Streptococcus mutans. J Contemp Dent Pract. 2012 Jan 1;13(1):71-4. doi: 10.5005/jp-journals-10024-1098. PMID: 22430697.
12. Galvão LC, Furletti VF, Bersan SM, da Cunha MG, Ruiz AL, de Carvalho JE, Sartoratto A, Rehder VL, Figueira GM, Teixeira Duarte MC, Ikegaki M, de Alencar SM, Rosalen PL. Antimicrobial Activity of Essential Oils against Streptococcus mutans and their Antiproliferative Effects. Evid Based Complement Alternat Med. 2012;2012:751435. doi: 10.1155/2012/751435. Epub 2012 May 24. PMID: 22685486; PMCID: PMC3368214.
13. Philip N, Walsh LJ. Cranberry Polyphenols: Natural Weapons against Dental Caries. Dent J (Basel). 2019 Mar 1;7(1):20. doi: 10.3390/dj7010020. PMID: 30823634; PMCID: PMC6473364.
14. Akhlaghi M, Ghasemi Nasab M, Riasatian M, Sadeghi F. Soy isoflavones prevent bone resorption and loss, a systematic review and meta-analysis of randomized controlled trials. Crit Rev Food Sci Nutr. 2020;60(14):2327-2341. doi: 10.1080/10408398.2019.1635078. Epub 2019 Jul 10. PMID: 31290343.
15. Iwasaki M, Sato M, Yoshihara A, Saito T, Kitamura K, Ansai T, Nakamura K. A 5-year longitudinal association between dietary fermented soya bean (natto) intake and tooth loss through bone mineral density in postmenopausal women: The Yokogoshi cohort study. Gerodontology. 2021 Sep;38(3):267-275. doi: 10.1111/ger.12523. Epub 2021 Jan 4. PMID: 33393717.
16. Gomes C, Martinho FC, Barbosa DS, Antunes LS, Póvoa HCC, Baltus THL, Morelli NR, Vargas HO, Nunes SOV, Anderson G, Maes M. Increased Root Canal Endotoxin Levels are Associated with Chronic Apical Periodontitis, Increased Oxidative and Nitrosative Stress, Major Depression, Severity of Depression, and a Lowered Quality of Life. Mol Neurobiol. 2018 Apr;55(4):2814-2827. doi: 10.1007/s12035-017-0545-z. Epub 2017 Apr 28. PMID: 28455694.
17. Aloutaibi YA, Alkarim AS, Qumri EM, Almansour LA, Alghamdi FT. Chronic Endodontic Infections and Cardiovascular Diseases: Does the Evidence Support an Independent Association? Cureus. 2021 Nov 24;13(11):e19864. doi: 10.7759/cureus.19864. PMID: 34976491; PMCID: PMC8712192.
18. Hyesook Kim, Hee Jung Lee, Ji-Yun Hwang, Eun-Hee Ha, Hyesook Park, Mina Ha, Ja Hyeong

Kim, Yun-Chul Hong, Namsoo Chang, Blood Cadmium Concentrations of Male Cigarette Smokers Are Inversely Associated with Fruit Consumption, The Journal of Nutrition, Volume 140, Issue 6, June 2010, Pages 1133–1138, https://doi.org/10.3945/jn.109.120659

# Heartburn, Ulcers, Nausea, and Vomiting

Collin Gow, C.N.C.
12/19/2021

The gastrointestinal ailments and symptoms in the title are all related and go hand-in-hand, which is why I have grouped them all together on the same education sheet. This article is a product of needing to do research for a client I am consulting on the above issues. I am writing it in a case study format on a client whom has been experiencing nausea and vomiting with increased frequency as time has gone on over the course of about 1 year. The subject is a middle-aged female with Type A blood, European ancestry, a history of ear infections/ear inflammation, a previous episode of severe dehydration during pregnancy 5.5 years ago, pineapple and honey allergies, and unremarkable CBC results as of late. Subject is otherwise considered generally healthy, with a generally healthy diet, and is someone who takes a few dietary supplements from time to time, including probiotics occasionally. She has had no feeling of burning in the esophagus, which is typical of heartburn/acid reflux. Besides nausea and vomiting, she has reported burping often and recently reported a "weird" taste in her mouth. The cause of the nausea and vomiting eluded both of us for some time due to very limited, emergency type visits that consisted of managing the nausea and vomiting while it was happening, limited information given by her upon questioning, and due to the symptoms only coming on occasionally in the past. Nevertheless, a number of educated guesses and approaches were tried for the nausea and vomiting, with limited success. Charcoal, ginger, *Saccharomyces boulardii,* Pepto Bismol (for bismuth) Dramamine, and peppermint were tried once she was already vomiting. Dramamine seemed to work the best. The vomiting would usually take about 4 hours to get over after initial onset and after a remedy was given. Going vegetarian helped to reduce the frequency of episodes for a few months, but more frequent symptoms resurfaced again. Cutting down foods inappropriate for her blood type did not do enough either. She was already avoiding some common allergens such as peanuts, wheat, and shellfish for years prior to when her problem appeared. While symptoms came and went, other than as-needed interventions, we mainly discussed foods to eat and foods to avoid to try to reduce the frequency of her episodes. We also discussed diagnostic tests to get and the many causes of nausea and vomiting. We thought in her case that it might be dehydration, or headaches, or otitis, or indigestion, or gastroparesis, or stress and anxiety, or maybe a hormonal imbalance that was triggering her issue. The only "preventive" supplements we tried throughout her trials were an encapsulated formula consisting of ginger, artichoke, and apple cider vinegar, in addition to feverfew capsules. The minor regimen seemed to help for a few weeks, but sure enough, the problems came back. We had not really tried many supplements or herbal remedies for the issue until 3 days ago when the situation came to a head. The nausea and vomiting began to appear daily and the subject went to a Walk-In clinic 3 days ago. No real diagnostic tests were run at the Walk-In. The visit consisted of talking to the doctor and the doctor reflecting back to my client the same hunches we already had going in. Prior to going in, we both came to the realization that the cause of it was probably due to silent heartburn and peptic ulcers caused by H. pylori. The doctor's diagnosis was "Frequent Nausea/Vomiting due to Significant Acid Reflux (sets of nausea reflex)" and Ondansetron, Omeprazole (a PPI), and Pepcid were prescribed. The subject preferred to go a natural route, however, so that is what we decided upon instead of prescription medication. With the ailments coming to a boiling point, the subject became interested in a more earnest approach than before, so we are now undertaking a serious regimen that we began the day of going to the Walk-In clinic. It includes supplements, foods, and lifestyle recommendations and we are laboring under the fairly confident assumption that the source of the symptoms is probably due to silent heartburn and peptic ulcers, along with H. pylori infection. So far, after 3 days on the regimen and under my relatively constant care and guidance, no nausea nor vomiting have occurred. While we are not out of the woodwork yet, I felt it pertinent to finish and publish this article for educational purposes. A number of the remedies in my protocol for the described client are listed on this sheet. If you (and/or someone you know) have been suffering from a severe case of mysterious nausea and vomiting that you (and/or a practitioner) have not been able to pinpoint the source of, you will find this article useful and helpful. However, even if you do not have heartburn or an ulcer or H. pylori infection, it will be most informative, and it may help you to connect the dots on other health challenges, especially those related to nausea and vomiting. For more information or further guidance via consultation on these issues, contact collingowcnc@gmail.com or collingowcnc@protonmail.com.

## Heartburn

Between 25% and 44% of people experience heartburn once a month. Heartburn may cause nocturnal hyperhydrosis (night sweats) and may be a cause of sleep apnea. I use the term heartburn instead of acid reflux, being that acid reflux more closely resembles a medical condition, and this article is not an attempt to treat, diagnose, or prevent any disease or condition. One should always talk to their practitioner before making any changes.

Signs and Symptoms: burning chest pain, regurgitation of fluid or food, trouble swallowing, cough, bronchospasms, hoarseness, sour taste in the back of the mouth, eroded enamel. Only a small percentage of heartburn events are symptomatic.

Causes and risk factors: H. pylori, peptic ulcer, smoking, insufficient exercise, anxiety and depression, high BMI, older age, poor food choice, defective peristalsis/gastroparesis, hypochlorhydria, gall stones, alcohol consumption, hiatal hernia, calcium deficiency, thyroid conditions, and pernicious anemia.

Complications of hypochlorhydria: folate, B12, calcium, magnesium, potassium, zinc, and iron deficiency, osteoporosis, SIBO.

Foods to avoid: carbonated beverages, coffee, alcohol, chocolate, mint, high fat foods, eating late at night, eating large meals, eating calorically dense meals, high protein foods, milk, sweets, and tomatoes.[1,2]

Foods to eat: vegetarian diet, vegetables, kiwi fruit, seaweed, okra, fiber, and non-citrus fruits.[2]

Lifestyle: get exercise, get enough sleep, walk after meals, and don't: smoke, drink strong alcohol, stress, do night work.[2]

Conventional treatments: PPIs, antibiotics. PPIs may decrease the absorption of vitamins and alkaline minerals, cause gut dysbiosis, SIBO, rebound stomach acid hypersecretion, increased reflux-like symptoms, and hypergastrinemia. Hypergastrinemia may be associated with an increased risk of stomach tumors.

Natural remedies: *Cydionia oblonga* (common quince), *Myrtus communis* (common myrtle),[3] *Optunia ficus-indica* (prickly pear) with olive leaf extract,[4] melatonin,[5] Bifidobacterium bifidum and Lactobacillus gasseri and other Bifidobacteria and Lactobacilli (GERD, regurgitation, heartburn, dyspepsia, nausea, abdominal pain, belching, gurgling, burping, vomiting),[6] *Aloe vera*.[7] Also, apple cider vinegar, Swedish bitters, DGL, slippery elm, licorice, marshmallow, fiber, d-limonene, alginic acid, zinc carnosine, bifidobacteria, Lactobacillus bulgaricus, vitamin E, vitamin A, gamma oryzanol, bentonite clay, neem leaf, barberry, cinnamon, goldenseal, dill, MSM, and a b-complex may be beneficial.

## Ulcers

Peptic ulcer: a discontinuation in the inner lining of the GI tract. It may occur in the stomach, duodenum, lower esophagus, and/or jejunum.

Signs and Symptoms:

- Epigastric pain within 15-30 mins after eating a meal for a gastric (stomach) ulcer or 2–3 hours after a meal for a duodenal ulcer. Nighttime pain is more common with duodenal ulcer.
- Bloating
- Abdominal fullness
- Nausea and vomiting
- Weight loss/weight gain
- Hematemesis (vomiting blood)
- Melena (dark feces due to partly digested blood)
- Difficulty swallowing
- Anemia

Some patients with ulcers have no symptoms.

Causes: H. pylori is the main cause. It causes 90% of duodenal ulcers and 70%–90% of gastric ulcers.[8] It colonizes 45–50% of people's stomachs worldwide and can lead to gastritis and stomach cancer as well. It is ranked as a Class I carcinogen by the WHO.[9] H. pylori infection may be one of the causes of Guillain-Barre Syndrome and it may be associated with an increased risk of blood clotting. Other causes include NSAIDS, medications, stress, cancer, viral infection such as CMV, cigarette smoking, vascular insufficiency, radiation, chemotherapy, Crohn's disease, Zollinger-Ellison syndrome, and hyper or hypochlorhydria (high or low stomach acid).

Diagnosis:

- Esophagogastroduodenoscopy
- Barium swallow
- H. pylori testing via either antibody testing, urea breath test, stool antigen test, urine-based ELISA and rapid urine test, or endoscopic biopsy
- CBC including liver function and amylase and lipase levels
- Epigastric tenderness upon physical exam
- Pancreatitis may be checked for with a CT scan
- Chest X-ray may be obtained to rule out other causes of chest pain

Natural remedies: One study showed that d-limonene pre-treatment had a 93%–100% inhibition of ethanol-induced ulcers in rats. Another study showed that d-limonene healed acetic acid-induced gastric ulcers in rats 56.2% better than controls.[10]

Natural compounds showing efficacy against H. pylori: garlic containing allicin, curcumin, mastic gum, cranberry, ginger. These last 3 may be more effective in vivo (in the body) than the others.[11] Also effective in vivo: *Strychnos pseudoquina*, *Qualea parviflora*, *Hancornia speciosa*, *Byrsonima intermedia*. Essential oils effective in vivo: *Cymbopogon citratus* (lemon grass). Essential oils effective in vitro: Mediterranean cypress, common Juniper, tea tree, lemon verbena, basil, peppermint, marjoram, thyme, oregano, sage, eucalyptus, *Ravensara aromatica*, lemon, lavender, common myrtle, Citrus lemon Burm. Rutaceae (Sicilian lemon) (contains high levels of limonene).[12,13] Others: Ceylon cinnamon, coriander, *Corydalis yanhusuo*, cumin, true cardamom, cloves, *Fritillaria thunbergii*, *Grindellia inuloides*, Bitter kola, four o'clock flower, olive leaf, oregano, plantain, rosemary, sage, thyme, broadleaf plantain (grows wild in Florida), *Terminalia chebula* (found in Triphala).[13] In addition, black seed, vitamin C, olive leaf, grapefruit seed extract, Lactobacillus rhamnosus, licorice, Lactobacillus reuteri, Bifidobacteria lactis, Bifidobacteria bifidus, and Lactobacillus acidophilus may all suppress or kill H. pylori.

Foods to eat: broccoli sprouts

## Nausea

Nausea is an unpleasant sensation that can precede vomiting.

Common causes of nausea[14]:

- Medications and toxic etiologies
- Disorders of the gut and peritoneum
- Cancer chemotherapy Mechanical obstruction
- Analgesics
- Gastric outlet obstruction
- Cardiovascular medications
- Small bowel obstruction
- Digoxin
- Functional gastrointestinal disorders
- Antiarrhythmics
- Functional dyspepsia
- Antihypertensives
- Chronic idiopathic nausea
- β-Blockers
- Cyclic Vomiting Syndrome
- Calcium-channel antagonists
- Idiopathic vomiting
- Hormonal preparations/therapies
- Oral antidiabetics
- Non-ulcer dyspepsia
- Oral contraceptives
- Irritable bowel syndrome
- Antibiotics/antivirals
- Organic gastrointestinal disorders
- Erythromycin
- Pancreatic adenocarcinoma
- Tetracycline
- Peptic ulcer disease
- Sulfonamides
- Cholecystitis
- Antituberculous drugs
- Pancreatitis
- Acyclovir
- Hepatitis
- Gastrointestinal medications
- Crohn's disease
- Sulfasalazine
- Neuromuscular disorders of the gastrointestinal tract
- Azathioprine
- Gastroparesis
- Nicotine
- Post-operative nausea and vomiting
- CNS active
- Chronic intestinal pseudo-obstruction
- Narcotics
- Antiparkinsonian drugs
- Migraine
- Anticonvulsants
- Increased intracranial pressure
- Malignancy
- Radiation therapy
- Hemorrhage

- Infarction
- Ethanol abuse
- Abscess
- Meningitis
- Congenital malformation
- Gastroenteritis
- Hydrocephalus
- Otitis media
- Pseudotumor cerebri
- Acute intermittent porphyria
- Seizure disorders
- Demyelinating disorders
- Psychiatric disease
- Cardiac disease
- Psychogenic vomiting
- Myocardial infarction
- Anxiety disorders
- Congestive heart failure
- Depression
- Radiofrequency ablation
- Pain
- Starvation
- Eating disorders
- Labyrinthine disorders
- Motion sickness
- Labyrinthitis
- Tumors
- Meniere's disease
- Iatrogenic causes
- Pregnancy
- Uremia
- Diabetic ketoacidosis
- Hyperparathyroidism
- Hypoparathyroidism
- Hyperthyroidism
- Addison's disease
- Infection

## Vomiting

Vomiting, aka "emesis" is "the forceful retrograde expulsion of gastric contents from the body"[15]. easier to fix than nausea. Vomiting can cause dehydration, metabolic alkalosis, and hypokalemia (low potassium).

<u>Conditions associated with Nausea *and* Vomiting[15]</u>:

- Toxic/metabolic
- Drugs, chemical toxins (alcohol, narcotics, digitalis glycosides)
- Biologic toxins (staphylococcal enterotoxin)
- Pregnancy (estrogens)
- Uremia
- Acidosis/ketosis (diabetic ketoacidosis, alcoholic ketosis)
- Electrolyte abnormalities (acute adrenal insufficiency, hypercalcemia)
- Infectious
- Viral infections
- Sepsis
- Meningitis/encephalitis
- Central nervous system
- Increased intracranial pressure (trauma, stroke, meningitis, malignant hypertension, vascular headache)
- Idiopathic epilepsy
- Vertigo/motion sickness
- Gastrointestinal
- Anatomic obstruction or motility disorder
    - Gastric outlet obstruction (peptic ulcer, carcinoma)
    - Small bowel obstruction (adhesion, herniation)
    - Colonic obstruction (carcinoma, volvulus)
    - Cholecystitis
    - Idiopathic pseudoobstruction
    - Diabetic gastroenteropathy
    - Inflammatory
    - Gastritis/duodenitis/peptic ulcer disease
    - Pancreatitis/hepatitis
    - Peritonitis/mesenteric ischemia
- Renal
- Renal colic

- Uremia
- Gynecologic
- Pregnancy
- Premenstrual stress syndrome
- Neoplasm
- Cardiopulmonary
- Inferior myocardial infarction
- Congestive heart failure
- Pulmonary embolism
- Post-tussive
- Psychogenic
- Anorexia nervosa/bulimia
- Chronic vomiting not associated with eating disorders

Rx drugs and OTC drugs used to treat vomiting: muscarinic receptor antagonists, histamine receptor antagonists, phenothiazines and dopamine receptor antagonists, 5-$HT_3$ receptor antagonists, $neurokinin_1$ receptor antagonists, anticholinergics, corticosteroids, 5-$HT_{1A}$ drugs, $GABA_B$ drugs, $CB_1$ receptor agonists.

Natural anti-emetics (anti-vomiting): ginger,[16] CBD, CBDA, and THC,[17,18] spearmint and peppermint,[19] Ceylon cinnamon and karanda fruits,[20] mango stem bark, leaves, and fruit and African black pepper fruits, leaves, and seeds,[21] *Allium sativum* (garlic) seeds, *Amomum cardamomum* (true cardamom) seeds, *Angelica archangelica* roots, fruit, and seeds, neem bark and flowers, *Achillea millefolium* (common yarrow) whole plant, Berberis vulgaris (European barberry) whole plant, *Calendula officinalis* florets, *Cinnamomum verum* fruits, Cinnamomum cassia whole plant, coriander fruits and leaves (juice), cumin fruits, amla fruits boiled in water, Hibiscus *rosa-sinensis* (Chinese hibiscus) whole herb, *Jasminum officinale* (common jasmine) whole plant, *Jatropha gossypifolia* (Bellyache bush) roots and leaves, *Ocimum basilicum* (basil) flowers, *Oryza sativa* (rice) fruits, *Panax ginseng* (Korean or Chinese ginseng) and *Panax quinquefolium* (American ginseng) roots, black pepper fruits, *Prunella vulgaris* (self-heal/heal-all), bloodroot roots, *Tinospora cordifolia* stem, stinging nettle leaves, grouseberry leaves, bog cranberry whole plant, and valerian roots.[22] *Nigella sativa* (black seed), Zataria multiflora, Bidens pilosa (Spanish needles), and carvacrol are natural $H_1$ receptor antagonists and have been used traditionally to stop vomiting.[23,24] Iberogast has been shown to have comparable effects to prescription 5-HT3 and 5-HT4 antagonists in functional gastrointestinal diseases.[25] American ginseng extract acts as an antagonist of the 5-HT3A receptor, which is involved in nausea and vomiting.[26] The medicinal plants Scutellaria baicalensis (Chinese Skullcap) roots, Korean red ginseng, American ginseng berry, Ganoderma lucidum, Zingiber officinale, grape seed extract, and the oil of Mentha spicata (spearmint) are reported to be effective in the treatment of nausea and vomiting, mostly in preclinical studies.[26]

Anti-emetic plants used in different parts of the world[22]:
Plant Family Part(s) used Country
Abrus precatorius Linn. Fabaceae Seeds China (Ahmed et al., 2013)
Abutilon indicum (L.) Sweet. Malvaceae Bark (juice) India (Ahmed et al., 2013)
Acacia farnesiana (L.) Willd. Mimosoideae Bangladesh (Hossan et al., 2009)
Acalypha fimbriata Schumach. & Thonn. Euphorbiaceae Leaves and stem Africa (Ajibesin et al., 2008)
Acalypha indica Linn. Leaves India (Rameshkumaret al., 2013)
Acalypha wilkesiana cv. godseffiana Muell Arg. Leaves and stem Africa (Akinyemi et al., 2005)
Achyranthes aspera Linn. Amaranthaceae Whole plant Pakistan (Ahmad, 2007) Seeds (tea) Pakistan (Qureshi et al., 2010)
Achillea millefolium Linn. Asteraceae Whole plant India (Ahmed et al., 2013)
Aconitum heterophyllumWall. ex Royle. Ranunculaceae Tubers Pakistan (Hazrat et al., 2011) Roots Pakistan (Gorsi and Miraj, 2002)

Aconitum palmatum D. Don. Roots India (Ahmed et al., 2013)
Acorus calamus L. Acoraceae Whole plant China (Motley, 1994)
Acorus gramineus Sol. ex Aiton Rhizome China (Ling et al., 2012)
Adenanthera pavonina Linn. Mimosoideae Leaves Africa (Holdsworth, 1977)
Adhatoda zeylanica Medic. Acanthaceae Whole plant India (Ahmed et al., 2013)
Aegle marmelos (L.) Correaex Roxb. Rutaceae Roots Nepal (Singh et al., 2012) India (Rasiya and Nayar, 2011)
Afzelia africana Sm. ex Pers. Fabaceae Aerial parts Africa (Ahmed et al., 2013)
Ageratum conyzoides Linn. Asteraceae Leaves (juice) New Guinea (Ahmed et al., 2013) India (Behera et al., 2006)
Ajuga bracteosa Wall. Labiatae Whole plant (powder cooked with cow's ghee) Pakistan (Ahmed et al., 2013)
Alhagi maurorum Medik. Fabaceae Whole plant India (Ahmed et al., 2013) Alhagi pseudalhagi(Bieb.) Desv.
Allium sativum L. (Garlic) Amaryllidaceae Seeds Palestine (Jaradat, 2005)
Alisma orientale (Sam.) Juz. Alismataceae Rhizomes China (Ahmed et al., 2013)
Allium humile Kunth. Liliaceae Leaves (chewing) Pakistan (Sher and Hussain, 2009)
Alpinia katsumadai Hayata. Zingiberaceae Seeds China (Ahmed et al., 2013)
Alpinia officinarum Hance. Rhizome China (Ahmed et al., 2013)
Alternanthera sessilis (L.) R. Br. Ex DC. Amaranthaceae Whole plant Pakistan (Arshad et al., 2011)
Amomum cardamomum Linn. (True cardamom) Zingiberaceae Seeds China (Ahmed et al., 2013)
Amomum globosum Lour. Fl. Cochinch. Seeds China (Ahmed et al., 2013)
Amomum kravanh Pire ex Gagnep. Fruits India (Ahmed et al., 2013) China (Ahmed et al., 2013)
Amomum tsao-koCrevost & Lemarié. Fruits and seeds China (Ahmed et al., 2013)
Amomum villosum Linn. Seeds China (Ahmed et al., 2013)
Amomum xanthioides Wall. Ex Baker. Fruits and seeds China (Ahmed et al., 2013)
Amorphophallus campanulatas (Roxb.) Blume ex Decne. Araceae Tuber India (Ahmed et al., 2013)

This is only a small portion of them. For an exhaustive list of plants visit...reference 22 below.

Other treatments showing efficacy: transcutaneous electroacupuncture (nausea and vomiting).[27]

References:


1. Newberry C, Lynch K. The role of diet in the development and management of gastroesophageal reflux disease: why we feel the burn. J Thorac Dis. 2019 Aug;11(Suppl 12):S1594-S1601. doi: 10.21037/jtd.2019.06.42. PMID: 31489226; PMCID: PMC6702398.
2. Zhang M, Hou ZK, Huang ZB, Chen XL, Liu FB. Dietary and Lifestyle Factors Related to Gastroesophageal Reflux Disease: A Systematic Review. Ther Clin Risk Manag. 2021 Apr 15;17:305-323. doi: 10.2147/TCRM.S296680. PMID: 33883899; PMCID: PMC8055252.
3. Salehi M, Karegar-Borzi H, Karimi M, Rahimi R. Medicinal Plants for Management of Gastroesophageal Reflux Disease: A Review of Animal and Human Studies. J Altern Complement Med. 2017 Feb;23(2):82-95. doi: 10.1089/acm.2016.0233. Epub 2016 Dec 20. PMID: 27996295.
4. Alecci U, Bonina F, Bonina A, Rizza L, Inferrera S, Mannucci C, Calapai G. Efficacy and Safety of a Natural Remedy for the Treatment of Gastroesophageal Reflux: A Double-Blinded Randomized-Controlled Study. Evid Based Complement Alternat Med. 2016;2016:2581461. doi: 10.1155/2016/2581461. Epub 2016 Oct 12. PMID: 27818697; PMCID: PMC5080480

5. Pereira Rde S. Regression of gastroesophageal reflux disease symptoms using dietary supplementation with melatonin, vitamins and aminoacids: comparison with omeprazole. J Pineal Res. 2006 Oct;41(3):195-200. doi: 10.1111/j.1600-079X.2006.00359.x. PMID: 16948779.
6. Kines K, Krupczak T. Nutritional Interventions for Gastroesophageal Reflux, Irritable Bowel Syndrome, and Hypochlorhydria: A Case Report. Integr Med (Encinitas). 2016 Aug;15(4):49-53. PMID: 27574495; PMCID: PMC4991651
7. Gao X, Liu J, Li L, Liu W, Sun M. A Brief Review of Nutraceutical Ingredients in Gastrointestinal Disorders: Evidence and Suggestions. Int J Mol Sci. 2020 Mar 6;21(5):1822. doi: 10.3390/ijms21051822. PMID: 32155799; PMCID: PMC7084955.
8. Malik TF, Gnanapandithan K, Singh K. Peptic Ulcer Disease. [Updated 2021 Jul 29]. In: StatPearls [Internet]. Treasure Island (FL): StatPearls Publishing; 2021 Jan-. Available from: https://www.ncbi.nlm.nih.gov/books/NBK534792/
9. Woolf A, Rose R. Gastric Ulcer. [Updated 2021 Jul 13]. In: StatPearls [Internet]. Treasure Island (FL): StatPearls Publishing; 2021 Jan-. Available from: https://www.ncbi.nlm.nih.gov/books/NBK537128/ Bonifácio BV, dos Santos Ramos MA, da Silva PB, Bauab TM. Antimicrobial activity of natural products against Helicobacter pylori: a review. Ann Clin Microbiol Antimicrob. 2014 Nov 19;13:54. doi: 10.1186/s12941-014-0054-0. PMID: 25406585; PMCID: PMC4243293.
10. Anandakumar, P., Kamaraj, S., & Vanitha, M. K. (2020). D-limonene: A multifunctional compound with potent therapeutic effects. Journal of Food Biochemistry. doi:10.1111/jfbc.13566 Cabbage juice.
11. Shmuely H, Domniz N, Yahav J. Non-pharmacological treatment of Helicobacter pylori. World J Gastrointest Pharmacol Ther. 2016 May 6;7(2):171-8. doi: 10.4292/wjgpt.v7.i2.171. PMID: 27158532; PMCID: PMC4848239.
12. Bonifácio BV, dos Santos Ramos MA, da Silva PB, Bauab TM. Antimicrobial activity of natural products against Helicobacter pylori: a review. Ann Clin Microbiol Antimicrob. 2014 Nov 19;13:54. doi: 10.1186/s12941-014-0054-0. PMID: 25406585; PMCID: PMC4243293.
13. Salehi B, Sharopov F, Martorell M, Rajkovic J, Ademiluyi AO, Sharifi-Rad M, Fokou PVT, Martins N, Iriti M, Sharifi-Rad J. Phytochemicals in Helicobacter pylori Infections: What Are We Doing Now? Int J Mol Sci. 2018 Aug 10;19(8):2361. doi: 10.3390/ijms19082361. PMID: 30103451; PMCID: PMC6121492.
14. Singh P, Yoon SS, Kuő B. Nausea: a review of pathophysiology and therapeutics. Therap Adv Gastroenterol. 2016 Jan;9(1):98-112. doi: 10.1177/1756283X15618131. PMID: 26770271; PMCID: PMC4699282.
15. Maule WF. Nausea and Vomiting. In: Walker HK, Hall WD, Hurst JW, editors. Clinical Methods: The History, Physical, and Laboratory Examinations. 3rd edition. Boston: Butterworths; 1990. Chapter 84. Available from: https://www.ncbi.nlm.nih.gov/books/NBK410/
16. Dudhatra GB, Mody SK, Awale MM, Patel HB, Modi CM, Kumar A, Kamani DR, Chauhan BN. A comprehensive review on pharmacotherapeutics of herbal bioenhancers. ScientificWorldJournal. 2012;2012:637953. doi: 10.1100/2012/637953. Epub 2012 Sep 17. PMID: 23028251; PMCID: PMC3458266.
17. Martínez V, Iriondo De-Hond A, Borrelli F, Capasso R, Del Castillo MD, Abalo R. Cannabidiol and Other Non-Psychoactive Cannabinoids for Prevention and Treatment of Gastrointestinal Disorders: Useful Nutraceuticals? Int J Mol Sci. 2020 Apr 26;21(9):3067. doi: 10.3390/ijms21093067. PMID: 32357565; PMCID: PMC7246936.
18. Yeasmin F, Choi HW. Natural Salicylates and Their Roles in Human Health. Int J Mol Sci. 2020

Nov 28;21(23):9049. doi: 10.3390/ijms21239049. PMID: 33260759; PMCID: PMC7731389. Xiao-Ban-Xia-Tang

19. Tayarani-Najaran Z., Talasaz-Firoozi E., Nasiri R., Jalali N., Hassanzadeh M. Antiemetic activity of volatile oil from Mentha spicata and Mentha x piperita in chemotherapy-induced nausea and vomiting. *Ecancermedicalscience*. 2013;7:290.
20. Dhatwalia J, Kumari A, Verma R, Upadhyay N, Guleria I, Lal S, Thakur S, Gudeta K, Kumar V, Chao JC, Sharma S, Kumar A, Manicum AE, Lorenzo JM, Amarowicz R. Phytochemistry, Pharmacology, and Nutraceutical Profile of Carissa Species: An Updated Review. Molecules. 2021 Nov 20;26(22):7010. doi: 10.3390/molecules26227010. PMID: 34834102; PMCID: PMC8624575.
21. Sofowora A, Ogunbodede E, Onayade A. The role and place of medicinal plants in the strategies for disease prevention. Afr J Tradit Complement Altern Med. 2013 Aug 12;10(5):210-29. doi: 10.4314/ajtcam.v10i5.2. PMID: 24311829; PMCID: PMC3847409.
22. Ahmed S, Hasan MM, Ahmed SW. Natural antiemetics: an overview. Pak J Pharm Sci. 2014 Sep;27(5 Spec no):1583-98. PMID: 25176254.
23. Keyhanmanesh R, Gholamnezhad Z, Boskabady MH. The relaxant effect of Nigella sativa on smooth muscles, its possible mechanisms and clinical applications. Iran J Basic Med Sci. 2014 Dec;17(12):939-49. PMID: 25859297; PMCID: PMC4387229.
24. Ahmad A, Husain A, Mujeeb M, Khan SA, Najmi AK, Siddique NA, Damanhouri ZA, Anwar F. A review on therapeutic potential of Nigella sativa: A miracle herb. Asian Pac J Trop Biomed. 2013 May;3(5):337-52. doi: 10.1016/S2221-1691(13)60075-1. PMID: 23646296; PMCID: PMC3642442.
25. Simmen U, Kelber O, Okpanyi SN, Jaeggi R, Bueter B, Weiser D. Binding of STW 5 (Iberogast) and its components to intestinal 5-HT, muscarinic M3, and opioid receptors. Phytomedicine. 2006;13 Suppl 5:51-5. doi: 10.1016/j.phymed.2006.03.012. Epub 2006 Sep 14. PMID: 16973340.
26. Haniadka R, Popouri S, Palatty PL, Arora R, Baliga MS. Medicinal plants as antiemetics in the treatment of cancer: a review. Integr Cancer Ther. 2012 Mar;11(1):18-28. doi: 10.1177/1534735411413266. Epub 2011 Aug 5. PMID: 21821652.
27. Chen JD, Yin J, Takahashi T, Hou X. Complementary and Alternative Therapies for Functional Gastrointestinal Diseases. Evid Based Complement Alternat Med. 2015;2015:138645. doi: 10.1155/2015/138645. Epub 2015 May 4. PMID: 26064152; PMCID: PMC4434213.

# Hypotension
# (Low Blood Pressure)

Low blood pressure may be caused by anemia, dehydration, heart failure, underactive thyroid, adrenal insufficiency/deficient glucocorticoid/mineralcorticoid secretion, diabetes, kidney problems such as diabetic nephropathy causing salt and albumin loss or chronic kidney disease, low blood volume due to decreased red blood cell mass, calcium deficiency, allergies, alcohol consumption, medications, infection, reduced baroreflex sensitivity, vascular stiffness, autonomic nervous system dysfunction, autonomic neuropathies, neurological conditions, multiple system atrophy, phenylalanine or tyrosine or noradrenaline deficiency, b-vitamin deficiency, Parkinson's, lack of venomotor tone, cholesterol deficiency, excessive amounts of the omega 6 arachidonic acid causing excessive vasodilatory prostaglandin synthesis i.e. inflammation, rheumatoid arthritis, and more. **Symptoms of low blood pressure are fatigue, brain fog, dizziness, light-headedness, fainting, nausea, and blurred vision**. I personally suffered from severe hypotension in the past and many of the nutraceuticals, herbs, and foods here have helped me.

**1. Greens Powders**—contain K1, magnesium, iron, and other blood building nutrients.

**2. Kelp and/or Spirulina**—Contain 52 or more minerals and boost thyroid function. The two highest sources of tyrosine in nature. Kelp is also high in iodine, which is the most important nutrient for thyroid health. Must take breaks from spirulina, since it contains B12 analogs.

**3. Whole Food Iron**—to build red blood cells. May be useful for anemia.

**4. Yohimbe**—adrenergic agonist that increases sympathetic nervous system tone and delays falls in blood pressure.[1]

**5. Butcher's Broom**—alpha-adrenergic agonist capable of tightening, toning, strengthening, and constricting peripheral blood vessels by stimulating the release of noradrenaline within the vascular wall to raise blood pressure. Takes a workload off the heart.[2]

**6. Phenylalanine and/or Tyrosine** and **Selenium**—help to create active thyroid hormones as well as adrenaline and dopamine.

**7. Hawthorn**—said to be helpful whether blood pressure is high or low. A good heart tonic for long term use for toning the heart.

**8. Licorice**—blocks the enzymes 11-ß-hydroxysteroid dehydrogenase type 2 and 5 ß-reductase, conferring mineralcorticoid-like effects and aldosterone-like effects, which helps the kidneys reabsorb sodium, while depleting potassium. These and/or other mechanisms may increase blood volume and raise blood pressure in some people, including people with diabetic nephropathy.[3,4] Good for adrenal insufficiency also. However, excess licorice intake can lead to pseudo-hyperaldosteronism.[3,4]

**9. Electrolytes** (sodium, chloride, potassium, calcium, magnesium)—for dehydration.

**10. Essential Amino Acids**—to make up for albumin loss.

**11. MSM**—may improve vascular stiffness.

**12. Astragalus**—to improve the function of the kidneys and adrenals.

References:


1. Verwaerde P, Tran MA, Montastruc JL, Senard JM, Portolan G. Effects of yohimbine, an alpha 2-adrenoceptor antagonist, on experimental neurogenic orthostatic hypotension. Fundam Clin Pharmacol. 1997;11(6):567-75. doi: 10.1111/j.1472-8206.1997.tb00862.x. PMID: 9444525.
2. Redman DA. Ruscus aculeatus (butcher's broom) as a potential treatment for orthostatic hypotension, with a case report. J Altern Complement Med. 2000 Dec;6(6):539-49. doi: 10.1089/acm.2000.6.539. PMID: 11152059.
3. Omar HR, Komarova I, El-Ghonemi M, Fathy A, Rashad R, Abdelmalak HD, Yerramadha MR, Ali Y, Helal E, Camporesi EM. Licorice abuse: time to send a warning message. Ther Adv Endocrinol Metab. 2012 Aug;3(4):125-38. doi: 10.1177/2042018812454322. PMID: 23185686; PMCID: PMC3498851.
4. Beretta-Piccoli C, Salvadé G, Crivelli PL, Weidmann P. Body-sodium and blood volume in a patient with licorice-induced hypertension. J Hypertens. 1985 Feb;3(1):19-23. doi: 10.1097/00004872-198502000-00004. PMID: 3889147.

# Joint Health

Collin Gow, C.N.C.

3/13/2022

**Joints are places where two bones meet**. They are complex structures consisting of ligaments, tendons, cartilage, synovial fluid, discs, surrounding muscles, and other tissues. Tissues and capsules of the joints are generally very high in collagen, hyaluronic acid, silica, manganese, sulfur, boron, calcium, and other nutrients. **Roughly 70% or 80% of the dry weight of ligaments and tendons is type 1 collagen.**[1,2] Histologically (microscopic, anatomical structurally) there are 3 types of joints—fibrous, cartilaginous, and synovial. Functionally, there are immoveable, slightly moveable, and freely moveable joints. **Cartilage is avascular** (contains no blood vessels) and some joints contain lymph nodes, such as the popliteal fossa of the knee.[3] **Muscle strength**, along with tendon strength, is especially important for the stability of synovial joints.[3] There are **360 joints** in the human body.[4] **Joint pain can be caused by trauma, infection, inflammation, autoimmune disease, genetic defects, aging, and cancer.**[5]

The following medicinal plants have been shown to have therapeutic potential for the joint disorders of osteoarthritis and rheumatoid arthritis: **Arnica montana (arnica), Boswellia spp. (boswellia), Curcuma spp. (turmeric), Equisetum arvense (horsetail), Harpagophytum procumbens (devil's claw), Salix spp. (white willow bark), Sesamum indicum (sesame), Symphytum officinalis (comfrey), Zingiber officinalis (ginger), Panax notoginseng (tienchi ginseng), and Whitania somnifera (ashwagandha).**[6] Horsetail is a great choice among these for joint strength, being that it is naturally high in silica. **Diatomaceous earth** and **bamboo** are also good sources of silica. Silica creates a mesh matrix which holds collagen together. **Tienchi ginseng** increases the proliferation and migration of ligament fibroblasts and the expression levels of collagen and fibronectin.[7] **Green tea, pomegranate peels, and grapeseed extract** inhibit and/or protect against collagenase in the body, an enzyme which leads to the destruction of the body's collagen. **Green tea, gotu kola**, and **Korean ginseng** stimulate the production of collagen. Dietary **omega 3s**, **vitamin K1**, and **K2** may also benefit osteoarthritis.[8] Omega 3s reduce pro-inflammatory compounds such as eicosanoids, reactive oxygen and nitrogen species, and cytokines, and they aid in the creation of anti-inflammatory compounds such as resolvins and protectins. Vitamin K mineralizes bones and cartilage. There is also good evidence that **avocado soybean unsaponifiables** are helpful for osteoarthritis and moderate evidence for **MSM**.[9] MSM is a type of sulfur. It is one of my personal favorites, especially for stiffness. **Hyaluronic acid** and glucosamine help build synovial fluid, which cushions and lubricates joints, reducing shock absorption. The Yuzurihara octogenarians of Japan have long life and beautiful, smooth, hydrated skin into their 80s, despite smoking, due to the hyaluronic acid content of their diets from fermented foods/potatoes. Hyaluronic acid can hold many times its weight in water. N-acetylglucosamine **(NAG)** (naturally high in insects, which is in the diets of many indigenous) acts as a precursor for the synthesis of hyaluronic acid. **Grapeseed extract** and **echinacea** work synergistically with hyaluronic acid; they inhibit the enzyme, hyaluronidase, which breaks down hyaluronic acid. Grapeseed extract also inhibits elastase, which breaks down elastin. Elastin is responsible for much of the load support of ligaments.[9] **Vitamin C** prevents the oxidation of collagen, and is essential for the hydroxylation of **lysine** and **proline**, which are necessary to synthesize collagen. **Glycine** is important for collagen synthesis also. **Chondroitin** is important for the health of chondrocytes, cells which maintain the cartilaginous matrix of the joints, which is composed of collagen and proteoglycans. **Copper** is necessary for the synthesis of collagen.

For the biosynthesis of collagen in my body, I more often prefer to provide the body with the nutrients that it uses to make collagen, versus consuming collagen itself. However, sometimes I do consume collagen and sometimes I consume a "vegan" collagen. When I consume regular, animal-based collagen, my sinuses get stuffed up, similar to eating a large portion of meat or dairy, but with a more marked effect than meat or dairy. In addition to mucus formation, excess animal foods tend to increase inflammation in the body as well, due to arachidonic acid and endotoxins. Yet, animal foods are necessary to consume in the diet (in the proper proportion), in my opinion.

I recommend picking 4 or 5 of the dietary supplements above and or trying to get them through the diet. Here are some joint healthy foods: high antioxidant/antiinflammatory, whole, raw, organic plant foods/beverages such as **sumac, cloves, allspice, Mexican oregano, mint, rosemary, sage, thyme, and cinnamon; berries, avocados, citrus, pomegranates, pineapple, papaya, and grapes; beets, Brussels sprouts, asparagus, onions, garlic, and red peppers; walnuts and black sesame seeds; hibiscus, nettle, and matcha tea; dark chocolate, espresso, and coffee; dog rose and dog rose hips; and black rice**. **Bamboo shoots** are good as well (for silica). Oats and beer are also high in silica, but I don't generally recommend those. Limit animal foods, focus on a plant dominant diet, yet consume fish and insects more often than turkey and beef. Organ meats in small quantities are okay. Mussels in small amounts are okay. Remember to **hydrate** and consume electrolytes as well. The nucleus pulposus of the intervetebral discs of the spine consist of as much as 86% water.[10]

References:


1. Henninger HB, Valdez WR, Scott SA, Weiss JA. Elastin governs the mechanical response of medial collateral ligament under shear and transverse tensile loading. Acta Biomater. 2015 Oct;25:304-12. doi: 10.1016/j.actbio.2015.07.011. Epub 2015 Jul 7. PMID: 26162584; PMCID: PMC4629914.
2. Hudson DM, Archer M, Rai J, Weis M, Fernandes RJ, Eyre DR. Age-related type I collagen modifications reveal tissue-defining differences between ligament and tendon. Matrix Biol Plus. 2021 Jun 2;12:100070. doi: 10.1016/j.mbplus.2021.100070. PMID: 34825162; PMCID: PMC8605237.
3. Juneja P, Munjal A, Hubbard JB. Anatomy, Joints. [Updated 2021 Jul 26]. In: StatPearls [Internet]. Treasure Island (FL): StatPearls Publishing; 2022 Jan-. Available from: https://www.ncbi.nlm.nih.gov/books/NBK507893/
4. Takiyama K, Yokoyama H, Kaneko N, Nakazawa K. Speed-dependent and mode-dependent modulations of spatiotem-poral modules in human locomotion extracted via tensor decom-position. Sci Rep. 2020 Jan 20;10(1):680. doi: 10.1038/s41598-020-57513-w. Erratum in: Sci Rep. 2020 Mar 6;10(1):4514. PMID: 31959831; PMCID: PMC6971295.
5. Havelin J, King T. Mechanisms Underlying Bone and Joint Pain. Curr Osteoporos Rep. 2018 Dec;16(6):763-771. doi: 10.1007/s11914-018-0493-1. PMID: 30370434; PMCID: PMC6554716.
6. Dragos D, Gilca M, Gaman L, Vlad A, Iosif L, Stoian I, Lupescu O. Phytomedicine in Joint Disorders. Nutrients. 2017 Jan 16;9(1):70. doi: 10.3390/nu9010070. PMID: 28275210; PMCID: PMC5295114.
7. Yu L, Xie J, Xin N, Wang Z. Panax notoginseng saponins promote wound repair of anterior cruciate ligament through phosphorylation of PI3K, AKT and ERK. Int J Clin Exp Pathol. 2015 Jan 1;8(1):441-9. PMID: 25755732; PMCID: PMC4348819.
8. Thomas S, Browne H, Mobasheri A, Rayman MP. What is the evidence for a role for diet and nutrition in osteoarthritis? Rheumatology (Oxford). 2018 May 1;57(suppl_4):iv61-iv74. doi:

10.1093/rheumatology/key011. PMID: 29684218; PMCID: PMC5905611.

9. Ameye LG, Chee WS. Osteoarthritis and nutrition. From nutraceuticals to functional foods: a systematic review of the scientific evidence. Arthritis Res Ther. 2006;8(4):R127. doi: 10.1186/ar2016. PMID: 16859534; PMCID: PMC1779427.
10. Waxenbaum JA, Reddy V, Futterman B. Anatomy, Back, Intervertebral Discs. [Updated 2021 Aug 10]. In: StatPearls [Internet]. Treasure Island (FL): StatPearls Publishing; 2022 Jan-. Available from: https://www.ncbi.nlm.nih.gov/books/NBK470583

# Leaky Gut

Collin Gow, C.N.C.

3/16/2022

**1. Butyrate** is the #1 product I would recommend for leaky gut. Butyrate is a short-chain fatty acid metabolite, aka "postbiotic", produced from the fermentation of fiber by gut microbiota. It's the primary source of energy for colon cells, supports normal intestinal PH, assists in modulating innate immunity, upregulates the expression of tight-junction proteins occludin and zonula occluden protein-1 (so does **Zinc**), and supports intestinal mucosa homeostasis. There are many studies on butyrate in the medical literature showing benefit for mechanisms that reduce "intestinal hyperpermeability" (leaky gut), plus it's great for the brain too. It has over 40 clinically documented therapeutic affects on the body. Start with 1 delayed release capsule, two times per day and work your way up to as many as 2 delayed release capsules, 3 times per day. Make sure you space out the capsules over the course of the day and make sure you consume a higher fiber diet if you get into the higher doses of butyrate.

**2. Boswellia** is anti-inflammatory, antimicrobial (antibacterial, antifungal, and antiviral), anti-histamine, immunomodulatory, and may be useful for many inflammatory bowel diseases. **Turmeric**, **Ginger**, **Propolis**, or **vitamin A** are good as well. Take 2-3 softgels/capsules of Boswellia twice daily.

**3.** Take a **Prebiotic** in powder form such as acacia, inulin, XOS, FOS, artichoke, chicory, or a combination thereof. Prebiotics feed probiotics, which are important for leaky gut. Start with 1 teaspoon per day if using acacia. Start with much less if using XOS or FOS. Eat a variety of **High Fiber** foods in your diet as well.

**4.** Take a **Probiotic** with a variety of strains and species and eat **Fermented Foods**.

**5.** Consume **Bitter** foods/beverages/supplements such as pine bark, ginkgo, green tea, fruit peels, fruit leaves, Swedish bitters, low-dose triphala, dandelion greens, and so on. These will aid digestion and tone the tight-junctions. Flavonoids like **quercetin** promote the assembly of TJ proteins also.

**6.** Consume **Slippery**/mucilaginous foods/beverages/supplements such as slippery elm, marshmallow, aloe, licorice, bananas, okra, fruit pectins/fruit, and seaweed. These will soothe, coat, lubricate, and aid in healing the lining of the gut. Try brewing a tea with 1-2 teaspoons of slippery elm powder in it per day, for instance. **NAG** would work synergistically with any of these.

**7. Glutamine** fuels the villi of the gastrointestinal tract. Take 3 grams per day on an empty stomach in the morning. **Glycine, Lysine, Proline,** and **Threonine** are beneficial amino acids for the gut as well. **Amla** or **Camu Camu** and **Bamboo** or **Horsetail** (also bitter) or **Bentonite Clay** would work synergistically with these aminos.

**8. Avoid refined/processed foods** & some of the **common allergens**, including peanuts, egg whites, non-fermented soy, wheat/gluten, and cow-sourced dairy. However, **colostrum is beneficial**. It may protect tight junctions from heat stress. **Limit oats**, **MCT oil**, & **alcohol**. Don't consume a high fat or high glucose diet. **Soak/sprout** any grains, nuts, or seeds. Eat for your blood type.

# Polycythemia Vera

Collin Gow, C.N.C.
6/6/2021

**Polycythemia vera** is a relatively rare, myeloproliferative (too many blood cells being made by the bone marrow) disorder affecting around .004% of the population.[1,2] It is associated with an acquired, not inherited, ***JAK2 V617F* or *JAK2 exon 12* gene mutation** (in 90-95% of cases[3,4]) that causes the neoplastic proliferation of the hematopoietic progenitor cells including **elevated red blood cells, elevated white blood cells, and elevated platelets**. Elevated hematocrit (volume percentage of red blood cells), hemoglobin, d-dimer, fibrinogen, and globulin are common, and myelofibrosis, and/or acute myeloid leukemia may also be present. A concomitant increase in **blood viscosity and risk of thrombosis** (which can cause strokes) are PV's major complications.[4] **Symptoms** are related to this hyperviscosity and thrombosis, which impairs oxygen delivery, and may include **headache, dizziness, fatigue, insomnia, visual disturbances, pruritus (itching caused by histamine surge), malaise, tinnitus, paresthesia (burning in the hands, legs, arms, feet), erythromelalgia (pain in the hands and feet), abdominal pain (spleen pain), enlarged spleen, gastritis, loss of appetite, early satiety, weight loss, claudication, and bleeding.**[4,5] **Diagnosis** of PV is defined by the WHO as **Hemoglobin > 16.5 g/dL in men/Hemoglobin > 16.0 g/dL in women, or Hematocrit > 49% in men/Hematocrit > 48% in women**. In addition, diagnosis consists of a **bone marrow biopsy** showing hypercellularity for age with trilineage growth (panmyelosis) including prominent erythroid, granulocytic, and megakaryocytic proliferation with pleomorphic, mature, megakaryocytes (differences in size), plus the presence of one of the varieties of ***JAK2* mutations**. **Standard medical treatment** for PV consists of **phlebotomy** and **low-dose aspirin**[4] and/or a **cytoreductive agent** such as hydroxyurea, interferon alpha, or busulfan,[5] (other novel drugs include Ropeginterferon Alpha-2b, Givinostat, and Idasanutlin), however, these medications come with risks, toxicities, and side-effects[6,7,8,9,10,11] which may further complicate PV. Ruxolitinib, under the trade name Jakafi®, is a second-line therapy for PV which also comes with side-effects[12]. In light of these side-effects, it may be of benefit to seek natural alternatives. Yet, this article is not an attempt to treat, diagnose, prevent, or cure any disease or condition. Talk to your doctor before making any changes. **This article merely highlights nutraceuticals that research has shown to possibly be of help for complications related to PV.** It may also be beneficial to know/eliminate **potential contributing factors** to or associations with the development of PV/Myeloproliferative diseases such as **smoking,**[13] **radioactive strontium-90,**[14] **radioactive caesium-137,**[14] **petroleum/benzene,**[15] **CT scans,**[16] **high childhood household density,**[16] **low childhood socioeconomic status,**[16] **Crohn's disease,**[17] **being of Jewish descent,**[17] **being a poultry worker,**[15] **fine particulate matter in utero,**[18] **genetic variants/polymorphisms in the NAT2 gene responsible for metabolizing xenobiotics/drugs/foreign toxic substances/carcinogens in tobacco smoke (the slow acetylator type)**[19] **murine myeloproliferative leukemia virus,**[20] **Friend leukemia virus,**[21] and so on. This last piece of etiology is very interesting as alcohol consumption is actually inversely associated with risk of PV and may harm fast and intermediate acetylators more than slow acetylators.[16,22] Alcohol and apple cider vinegar contain high amounts of acetic acid. Perhaps the consumption of these would aid in the battle against PV by enhancing the detoxification of xenobiotics via their high acetic acid content? That being said, I'm not necessarily recommending that you go drink 5 beers every night and it's a wild guess that acetic acid would help slow acetylators. In addition, although PV occurs usually around the median age of 60 and is **generally considered an acquired, not inherited disease, familial clusters have been found (one study showing a 5-7 fold increased risk for first degree relatives),**[23,15] so it may be a good idea to have first degree relatives of a known PV patient tested for the genetic polymorphism.

**Natural anti-thrombotic alternatives to aspirin**: (according to Chris Kresser, aspirin increases the risk of bleeding, ulcer, H. pylori infection, G.I. damage, Crohn's, hearing loss, tinnitus, influenza mortality, and Reye's syndrome and some of these effects even occur taking low-dose aspirin[24])**:** cacao, omega 3s, ajoene in garlic, ginger, ginkgo, and vitamin E **(anti-platelet properties)**;[25,26,27,28] anise and dong quai **(anticoagulant effects)**; fucus **(heparin-like activity)**; danshen **(antithrombin III-like activity and anticoagulant bioavailability)**; vitamin E **(vitamin K antagonist activity)**;[28] IGF-1 **(increases nitric oxide synthase)**;[29] grapeseed extract **(antiplatelet and anticoagulant)**;[30] pycnogenol **(anti-platelet, increases NO, reduces endothelin-1)**;[31] nattokinase, serrapeptase, and lumbrokinase **(fibrinolytic) (be very careful with these)**;[32,33] plus black seed oil, evening primrose oil, quercetin, chrysin, resveratrol, thunder god root, prickly ash bark, and policosanol. A number of structural and functional platelet abnormalities exist in PV, however, and some of these anti-thrombotics may not address those abnormalities. Yet, being that aspirin can cause some of the same issues already present in PV, namely bleeding, tinnitus, and gastric issues, it would behoove one to pay attention to these natural alternatives. While bleeding time can be prolonged by some, but not all of these natural remedies too, at the very least, one may be eliminating the tinnitus and gastric side effects of aspirin by choosing a natural remedy. My nutritional intuition, developed over many years as a practitioner, leans towards combining either grapeseed extract or pycnogenol with one of the other alternatives above, due to their astringent quality, which may help to tone blood vessels. Ginkgo would be an obvious choice instead of these two, being that it is astringent, a JAK/STAT inhibitor, and is studied for tinnitus, yet some studies have shown it can prolong bleeding time. Yet, I still maintain that ginkgo may have less side effects than aspirin.

**Natural JAK/STAT pathway/signaling inhibitors** (STATs migrate toward the nucleus where they act as transcription factors, activating or repressing genes (such as JAK2) that are important in cell proliferation and survival;[34] down-regulation of the JAK/STAT pathway may be important for PV)**:** ginkgo,[35,36] sulforaphane and moringin (isolated from moringa),[37] blackberry, boysenberry, feijoa, pomegranate, rosehip, strawberry, genistein, and resveratrol,[38] bigelovin from the flower of the Chinese herb *Inula hupehensis*,[39] parthenolide from feverfew,[40] boswellic acid,[41] propolis,[42] plus thunder god root, saffron, fermented ginseng, honokiol, curcubitacin, and licorice. In addition to anti-thrombotics, inhibiting the JAK/STAT pathway may reduce the risk of thrombosis as well.[43,44]

**Natural Anti-inflammatories** (inflammation may exacerbate thrombogenesis in PV and elevated cytokine levels such as IL-11, IL-12, IL-13, IL-5, and IL-7 are present in people with PV[43,44,45]) (**spleen pain and feet pain** in PV may be worsened by inflammation)**:** nearly everything listed so far in this article is anti-inflammatory,[46-54] especially boswellia, ginger, quercetin, ginkgo, black seed oil, resveratrol, omega 3s, garlic, grapeseed extract, pycnogenol, and propolis, however, here's the proof, along with more natural products with anti-inflammatory compounds/effects: lavender, turmeric, licorice, *Cannabis*, *Artemisia*, cayenne, saffron, pumpkin, garlic, St. John's Wort, black seed, plantain, gotu kola, ashwagandha, ginger, nettle,[46] rosehips, boswellia, avocado soybean fraction,[47] cinnamon, black pepper, vitamin C, propolis, probiotics, quercetin,[48] aged garlic extract, alpha lipoic acid, niacin, nicotinamide,[49] green tea, cat's claw, pomegranate, bromelain, devil's claw,[50] ginkgo, rhubarb, resveratrol, berries, brassica family foods,[51] *Acanthopanax senticosus*, *Actinidia arguta*, *Ainsliaea fragrans Champ*, *Ampelopsis grossedentata*, *Cyperus rotundus*, *Dilodendron bipinnatum Radlk*, *Hibiscus sabdariffa*, *Lycium barbarum*, moringa, schisandra, smilax,[52] rosemary, borage, sage, basil, holy basil, black nightshade, cocklebur, red-bark oak, European barberry, amla, chamomile,[53] *Piper* *kadsura*, *Phyllanthus amarus*, *Achillea pannonica*, *Kigelia africana*, *Nyctanthes arbortristis*,[54] plus andrographis, tart cherry, white willow bark, hops, Chinese skullcap, olive fruit, olive leaf, clove, echinacea, oregano, thyme, primrose oil, black currant, bilberry, reishi, etc. Of course, some of these may not be appropriate for PV specifically. Anti-inflammatories are important also because **PV cells have an increased sensitivity to growth factors and cytokines** (inflammatory proteins released by cells). Anti-inflammatories have the potential to thin the blood, so one should be conscious of that when taking in conjunction with anti-thrombotics.

**Myelofibrosis:** danshen (*Salvia M.*).[55] Allogenic stem cell transplantation is considered the only cure for MF.[56]

**Pruritus** (anti-histamines)**:** boswellia, quercetin.

**Homeopathic phosphorus:** an unexpected long survival of a patient with PV who was treating himself with nearly nothing but homeopathic phosphorus exists in the medical literature.[57] This is quite interesting as the phosphorylation of STATs and JAK2 plays a key role in the pathogenesis of PV. Also, radioactive phosphorus has been used in the past for the treatment of PV. Lastly, adenosine diphosphate increases thrombin production in those with myeloproliferative neoplasms, defective expression of SHP-1 phosphatase has been found in people with PV, and increased protein tyrosine phosphatase activity in polycythemia vera cells has been demonstrated.[58,59,60] Clearly, something is going on with phosphorus in PV. Something is going on with valine, phenylalanine, and tyrosine as well being that the main JAK mutation in PV involves a substitution of valine with phenylalanine and Janus Kinase (JAK) is a tyrosine kinase (phenylalanine is a precursor to tyrosine in the body).

**Natural growth factor reducers:** black seed (FGF), Fritillaria thunbergii (IGF-1), garlic (thymidine, VEGF, FGF2), lycopene (IGF-1), quercetin (EGF, VEGF), parsley (VEGF), chili pepper (VEGF), curcumin (EGF, VEGF, bFGF), green tea (VEGF), resveratrol (FGF, VEGF), soy (FGF2, VEGF), vanilla bean (HGF), cloves (VEGF), sulforaphane (PDGF, VEGF), (Gupta, Kim, Aggarwal et al.), (Wargovich, Morris, Weber et al.), (Agbarya, Ruimi, Epelbaum...et al.).

**Links:** https://www.youtube.com/watch?v=BfFCAfT3zcc

**References**

1. Ma X, Vanasse G, Cartmel B, Wang Y, Selinger HA. Prevalence of polycythemia vera and essential thrombocythemia. Am J Hematol. 2008 May;83(5):359-62. doi: 10.1002/ajh.21129. PMID: 18181200.
2. Stein, Brady L et al. "Polycythemia Vera: An Appraisal of the Biology and Management 10 Years After the Discovery of JAK2 V617F." *Journal of clinical oncology : official journal of the American Society of Clinical Oncology* vol. 33,33 (2015): 3953-60. doi:10.1200/JCO.2015.61.6474
3. Pillai AA, Fazal S, Babiker HM. Polycythemia. [Updated 2021 Jan 29]. In: StatPearls [Internet]. Treasure Island (FL): StatPearls Publishing; 2021 Jan-. Available from: https://www.ncbi.nlm.nih.gov/books/NBK526081/
4. Lu X, Chang R. Polycythemia Vera. [Updated 2020 May 13]. In: StatPearls [Internet]. Treasure Island (FL): StatPearls Publishing; 2021 Jan-. Available from: https://www.ncbi.nlm.nih.gov/books/NBK557660/

5. Thapa B, Fazal S, Parsi M, et al. Myeloproliferative Neoplasms. [Updated 2020 Aug 13]. In: StatPearls [Internet]. Treasure Island (FL): StatPearls Publishing; 2021 Jan-. Available from: https://www.ncbi.nlm.nih.gov/books/NBK531464/
6. Kwok, Chun Shing, and Yoon K Loke. "Critical Overview on the Benefits and Harms of Aspirin." *Pharmaceuticals (Basel, Switzerland)* vol. 3,5 1491-1506. 14 May. 2010, doi:10.3390/ph3051491
7. Arif H, Aggarwal S. Salicylic Acid (Aspirin) [Updated 2020 Jul 13]. In: StatPearls [Internet]. Treasure Island (FL): StatPearls Publishing; 2021 Jan-. Available from: https://www.ncbi.nlm.nih.gov/books/NBK519032/
8. Agrawal, Rohit Kumar et al. "Hydroxyurea in sickle cell disease: drug review." *Indian journal of hematology & blood transfusion : an official journal of Indian Society of Hematology and Blood Transfusion* vol. 30,2 (2014): 91-6. doi:10.1007/s12288-013-0261-4
9. LiverTox: Clinical and Research Information on Drug-Induced Liver Injury [Internet]. Bethesda (MD): National Institute of Diabetes and Digestive and Kidney Diseases; 2012-. Hydroxyurea. [Updated 2018 Mar 26]. Available from: https://www.ncbi.nlm.nih.gov/books/NBK548724/
10. Nazha, Aziz, and Aaron T Gerds. "Where to Turn for Second-Line Cytoreduction After Hydroxyurea in Polycythemia Vera?." *The oncologist* vol. 21,4 (2016): 475-80. doi:10.1634/theoncologist.2015-0380
11. Alvarez-Larrán A, Martínez-Avilés L, Hernández-Boluda JC, Ferrer-Marín F, Antelo ML, Burgaleta C, Mata MI, Xicoy B, Martínez-Trillos A, Gómez-Casares MT, Durán MA, Marcote B, Ancochea A, Senín A, Angona A, Gómez M, Vicente V, Cervantes F, Bellosillo B, Besses C. Busulfan in patients with polycythemia vera or essential thrombocythemia refractory or intolerant to hydroxyurea. Ann Hematol. 2014 Dec;93(12):2037-43. doi: 10.1007/s00277-014-2152-7. Epub 2014 Jul 2. PMID: 24981691.
12. https://www.jakafi.com/myelofibrosis/side-effects
13. Hasselbalch HC. Smoking as a contributing factor for development of polycythemia vera and related neoplasms. Leuk Res. 2015 Sep 9:S0145-2126(15)30373-8. doi: 10.1016/j.leukres.2015.09.002. Epub ahead of print. PMID: 26463040.
14. IARC Working Group on the Evaluation of Carcinogenic Risks to Humans. Ionizing Radiation, Part 2: Some Internally Deposited Radionuclides. Lyon (FR): International Agency for Research on Cancer; 2001. (IARC Monographs on the Evaluation of Carcinogenic Risks to Humans, No. 78.) 3, Studies of Cancer in Experimental Animals. Available from: https://www.ncbi.nlm.nih.gov/books/NBK396557/
15. Gross-Davis, Carol Ann. "Environmental Etiology of Polycythemia Vera, Essential Thrombocythemia and Primary Myelofibrosis: A Case-Control Study in Northeast Pennsylvania." (2014).
16. Duncombe, Andrew S et al. "Modifiable Lifestyle and Medical Risk Factors Associated With Myeloproliferative Neoplasms." HemaSphere vol. 4,1 e327. 3 Jan. 2020, doi:10.1097/HS9.0000000000000327
17. Anderson LA, Duncombe AS, Hughes M, Mills ME, Wilson JC, McMullin MF. Environmental, lifestyle, and familial/ethnic factors associated with myeloproliferative neoplasms. Am J Hematol. 2012 Feb;87(2):175-82. doi: 10.1002/ajh.22212. Epub 2011 Nov 11. PMID: 22076943.
18. Bhattarai, Govinda et al. "Maternal exposure to fine particulate matter during pregnancy induces progressive senescence of hematopoietic stem cells under preferential impairment of the bone marrow microenvironment and aids development of myeloproliferative disease." Leukemia vol. 34,5 (2020): 1481-1484. doi:10.1038/s41375-019-0665-8
19. Gross-Davis, Carol Ann et al. "The role of genotypes that modify the toxicity of chemical mutagens in the risk for myeloproliferative neoplasms." International journal of environmental research and public health vol. 12,3 2465-85. 24 Feb. 2015, doi:10.3390/ijerph120302465

20. Wendling F, Varlet P, Charon M, Tambourin P. MPLV: a retrovirus complex inducing an acute myeloproliferative leukemic disorder in adult mice. Virology. 1986 Mar;149(2):242-6. doi: 10.1016/0042-6822(86)90125-x. PMID: 3004028.
21. Chu, Charles C et al. "Torque teno virus 10 isolated by genome amplification techniques from a patient with concomitant chronic lymphocytic leukemia and polycythemia vera." Molecular medicine (Cambridge, Mass.) vol. 17,11-12 (2011): 1338-48. doi:10.2119/molmed.2010.00110
22. Chen C, Ricks S, Doody DR, Fitzgibbons ED, Porter PL, Schwartz SM. N-Acetyltransferase 2 polymorphisms, cigarette smoking and alcohol consumption, and oral squamous cell cancer risk. Carcinogenesis. 2001 Dec;22(12):1993-9. doi: 10.1093/carcin/22.12.1993. PMID: 11751430.
23. Seaman, Vincent et al. "A multidisciplinary investigation of a polycythemia vera cancer cluster of unknown origin." International journal of environmental research and public health vol. 7,3 (2010): 1139-52. doi:10.3390/ijerph7031139
24. https://chriskresser.com/4-natural-alternatives-to-aspirin/
25. Rein D, Paglieroni TG, Wun T, Pearson DA, Schmitz HH, Gosselin R, Keen CL. Cocoa inhibits platelet activation and function. Am J Clin Nutr. 2000 Jul;72(1):30-5. doi: 10.1093/ajcn/72.1.30. PMID: 10871557.
26. Shafiekhani, Mojtaba et al. "Comparison of antiplatelet activity of garlic tablets with cardio-protective dose of aspirin in healthy volunteers: a randomized clinical trial." Avicenna journal of phytomedicine vol. 6,5 (2016): 550-557.
27. Marx, Wolfgang et al. "The Effect of Ginger (Zingiber officinale) on Platelet Aggregation: A Systematic Literature Review." *PloS one* vol. 10,10 e0141119. 21 Oct. 2015, doi:10.1371/journal.pone.0141119
28. Mousa SA. Antithrombotic effects of naturally derived products on coagulation and platelet function. Methods Mol Biol. 2010;663:229-40. doi: 10.1007/978-1-60761-803-4_9. PMID: 20617421.
29. McCarty MF. IGF-I activity may be a key determinant of stroke risk--a cautionary lesson for vegans. Med Hypotheses. 2003 Sep;61(3):323-34. doi: 10.1016/s0306-9877(02)00241-4. PMID: 12944100.
30. Bijak, Michal et al. "Dual Anticoagulant/Antiplatelet Activity of Polyphenolic Grape Seeds Extract." *Nutrients* vol. 11,1 93. 5 Jan. 2019, doi:10.3390/nu11010093
31. Nocun M, Ulicna O, Muchova J, Durackova Z, Watala C. French maritime pine bark extract Pycnogenol reduces thromboxane generation in blood from diabetic male rats. Biomed Pharmacother. 2008 Mar;62(3):168-72. doi: 10.1016/j.biopha.2007.07.002. Epub 2007 Jul 30. PMID: 17698319.
34. de Freitas, Renata Mendes, and Carlos Magno da Costa Maranduba. "Myeloproliferative neoplasms and the JAK/STAT signaling pathway: an overview." *Revista brasileira de hematologia e hemoterapia* vol. 37,5 (2015): 348-53. doi:10.1016/j.bjhh.2014.10.001
32. Adivitiya, and Yogender Pal Khasa. "The evolution of recombinant thrombolytics: Current status and future directions." *Bioengineered* vol. 8,4 (2017): 331-358. doi:10.1080/21655979.2016.1229718
33. Weng, Yunqi et al. "Nattokinase: An Oral Antithrombotic Agent for the Prevention of Cardiovascular Disease." *International journal of molecular sciences* vol. 18,3 523. 28 Feb. 2017, doi:10.3390/ijms18030523
35. Zhang, Yehao et al. "Ginkgo biloba Extract Inhibits Astrocytic Lipocalin-2 Expression and Alleviates Neuroinflammatory Injury via the JAK2/STAT3 Pathway After Ischemic Brain Stroke." *Frontiers in pharmacology* vol. 9 518. 16 May. 2018, doi:10.3389/fphar.2018.00518
36. Liang JR, Yang H. Ginkgolic acid (GA) suppresses gastric cancer growth by inducing apoptosis and suppressing STAT3/JAK2 signaling regulated by ROS. Biomed Pharmacother. 2020 May;125:109585. doi: 10.1016/j.biopha.2019.109585. Epub 2020 Feb 25. PMID: 32106377.
37. Michl, Carina et al. "The Chemopreventive Phytochemical Moringin Isolated from Moringa

oleifera Seeds Inhibits JAK/STAT Signaling." *PloS one* vol. 11,6 e0157430. 15 Jun. 2016, doi:10.1371/journal.pone.0157430
38. Martin, Harry & Burgess, Elaine & Smith, Wendy & Mcghie, Tony & Cooney, Janine & Lunken, Rona & Guzman, Erika & Trower, Tania & Perry, Nigel. (2014). JAK2 and AMP-kinase inhibition in vitro by food extracts, fractions and purified phytochemicals. Food & function. 6. 10.1039/c4fo00626g.
39. Zhang, Hao-hao et al. "Bigelovin inhibits STAT3 signaling by inactivating JAK2 and induces apoptosis in human cancer cells." Acta pharmacologica Sinica vol. 36,4 (2015): 507-16. doi:10.1038/aps.2014.143
40. Liu, Man et al. "Parthenolide Inhibits STAT3 Signaling by Covalently Targeting Janus Kinases." *Molecules (Basel, Switzerland)* vol. 23,6 1478. 19 Jun. 2018, doi:10.3390/molecules23061478
41. Kunnumakkara, Ajaikumar B et al. "Boswellic acid blocks signal transducers and activators of transcription 3 signaling, proliferation, and survival of multiple myeloma via the protein tyrosine phosphatase SHP-1." Molecular cancer research : MCR vol. 7,1 (2009): 118-28. doi:10.1158/1541-7786.MCR-08-0154
42. Okamoto Y, Tanaka M, Fukui T, Masuzawa T. Brazilian propolis inhibits the differentiation of Th17 cells by inhibition of interleukin-6-induced phosphorylation of signal transducer and activator of transcription 3. Immunopharmacol Immunotoxicol. 2012 Oct;34(5):803-9. doi: 10.3109/08923973.2012.657304. Epub 2012 Feb 9. PMID: 22316079.
43. Kroll, Michael H et al. "Mechanisms of thrombogenesis in polycythemia vera." *Blood reviews* vol. 29,4 (2015): 215-21. doi:10.1016/j.blre.2014.12.002
44. Cuthbert, Danielle, and Brady Lee Stein. "Polycythemia Vera-Associated Complications: Pathogenesis, Clinical Manifestations, And Effects On Outcomes." *Journal of blood medicine* vol. 10 359-371. 18 Oct. 2019, doi:10.2147/JBM.S189922
45. Hermouet, Sylvie et al. "Pathogenesis of Myeloproliferative Neoplasms: Role and Mechanisms of Chronic Inflammation." *Mediators of inflammation* vol. 2015 (2015): 145293. doi:10.1155/2015/145293
46. Dar, Khalid & Bhat, Aashiq & Amin, Shajrul & Masood, Akbar & Zargar, Mohammad & Ganie, Showkat. (2016). Inflammation: A Multidimensional Insight on Natural Anti-Inflammatory Therapeutic Compounds. Current medicinal chemistry. 23. 10.2174/0929867323666160817163531.
47. Chrubasik JE, Roufogalis BD, Chrubasik S. Evidence of effectiveness of herbal antiinflammatory drugs in the treatment of painful osteoarthritis and chronic low back pain. Phytother Res. 2007 Jul;21(7):675-83. doi: 10.1002/ptr.2142. PMID: 17444576.
48. Mrityunjaya, M et al. "Immune-Boosting, Antioxidant and Anti-inflammatory Food Supplements Targeting Pathogenesis of COVID-19." Frontiers in immunology vol. 11 570122. 7 Oct. 2020, doi:10.3389/fimmu.2020.570122
49. Takechi R, Pallebage-Gamarallage MM, Lam V, Giles C, Mamo JC. Nutraceutical agents with anti-inflammatory properties prevent dietary saturated-fat induced disturbances in blood-brain barrier function in wild-type mice. J Neuroinflammation. 2013 Jun 19;10:73. doi: 10.1186/1742-2094-10-73. PMID: 23782872; PMCID: PMC3693897.
50. Akhtar, Nahid, and Tariq M Haqqi. "Current nutraceuticals in the management of osteoarthritis: a review." Therapeutic advances in musculoskeletal disease vol. 4,3 (2012): 181-207. doi:10.1177/1759720X11436238
51. Andrade, Paula B, and Patrícia Valentão. "Insights into Natural Products in Inflammation." International journal of molecular sciences vol. 19,3 644. 25 Feb. 2018, doi:10.3390/ijms19030644
52. Arulselvan, Palanisamy et al. "Role of Antioxidants and Natural Products in

Inflammation." Oxidative medicine and cellular longevity vol. 2016 (2016): 5276130. doi:10.1155/2016/5276130
53. Yatoo, Dr. Mohammad & Gopalakrishnan, Arumugam & Saxena, Archana & Parray, Oveas & Tufani, Dr Noor & Chakraborty, Sandip & Tiwari, Ruchi & Dhama, Kuldeep & Iqbal, Hafiz. (2018). Anti-Inflammatory Drugs and Herbs with Special Emphasis on Herbal Medicines for Countering Inflammatory Diseases and Disorders - A Review. Recent Patents on Inflammation & Allergy Drug Discovery. 12. 10.2174/1872213X12666180115153635.
54. Beg, Sarwar et al. "Systematic review of herbals as potential anti-inflammatory agents: Recent advances, current clinical status and future perspectives." Pharmacognosy reviews vol. 5,10 (2011): 120-37. doi:10.4103/0973-7847.91102
55. Li, Jie et al. "Exploring the Mechanism of Danshen against Myelofibrosis by Network Pharmacology and Molecular Docking." *Evidence-based complementary and alternative medicine : eCAM* vol. 2018 8363295. 5 Dec. 2018, doi:10.1155/2018/8363295
56. Lee, Sung-Eun. "Disease modifying agents of myeloproliferative neoplasms: a review." *Blood research* vol. 56,S1 (2021): S26-S33. doi:10.5045/br.2021.2020325
57. Frass, Michael & Gaertner, Katharina. (2019). Unexpected Long Survival of a Patient with Polycythemia Vera. OBM Integrative and Complementary Medicine. 4. 1-1. 10.21926/obm.icm.1902023.
58. Zhao ZJ, Vainchenker W, Krantz SB, Casadevall N, Constantinescu SN. Role of tyrosine kinases and phosphatases in polycythemia vera. Semin Hematol. 2005 Oct;42(4):221-9. doi: 10.1053/j.seminhematol.2005.05.019. PMID: 16210035.
59. Wickrema A, Chen F, Namin F, Yi T, Ahmad S, Uddin S, Chen YH, Feldman L, Stock W, Hoffman R, Platanias LC. Defective expression of the SHP-1 phosphatase in polycythemia vera. Exp Hematol. 1999 Jul;27(7):1124-32. doi: 10.1016/s0301-472x(99)00043-0. PMID: 10390187.
60. Presseizen K, Friedman Z, Shapiro H, Radnay J, Ellis MH. Phosphatidylserine expression on the platelet membrane of patients with myeloproliferative disorders and its effect on platelet-dependent thrombin formation. Clin Appl Thromb Hemost. 2002 Jan;8(1):33-9. doi: 10.1177/107602960200800104. PMID: 11991237.

# Eating Food

# Collin Gow, C.N.C.'s True (Waterless) Nutrient Density Scale

Collin Gow, C.N.C.

3/13/2022

The following nutrient values were gathered and calculated from the **USDA's FoodData Central nutrient profile database**. It was accessed from April through May of 2018 to obtain and calculate this information. I was unsatisfied with both Dr. Joel Fuhrman's and Mathieu Lalonde's methods of calculating their nutrient density scales, so I wanted to investigate the data myself and make my own. What makes my nutrient density scale unique and a "true" nutrient density scale, in my eyes, is that I have subtracted water from all foods in order to put them on a level playing field. If, for instance, I'm comparing a dried herb or dried spice to a fresh herb or fresh spice, or to a watermelon for that matter, that is not a fair comparison, due to the vast differences in water content. Or if, for example, I'm comparing a beverage such as milk or juice or brewed coffee to a piece of meat or powdered milk, those also have huge differences in water content. As I spent over 90 hours examining, extracting, and calculating the data within the USDA's nutrient database, over and over it didn't make sense to not extract the water. I also did not allow processed "foods" to be on the list, since they aren't real, whole, unadulterated foods, and can therefore artificially climb the list because of additives. Plus, some processed foods you can't find in grocery stores. For instance, Taco Bell Boarder Sauce topped the list for "vitamin A", but I figured that had to be water-soluble forms of of vitamin A (carotenoids), which aren't the same as fat-soluble vitamin A, and you can't buy Taco Bell Boarder Sauce in a grocery store, as far as I know, nor would you want to, being that, besides having high "vitamin A" and probably high vitamin C, it probably isn't healthy in other ways. Plus, you can only eat so much of that, which should be factored in. Sure, Taco Bell Boarder Sauce (or some other processed food) might be very high in a particular nutrient per 100g, but if you consumed 100g of it, you'd probably be shitting your brains out. Nobody would or could ever consume that much of it at one time, so, overall, you actually don't end up getting much of the particular nutrient that it is high in, because you can only consume so much of it. That's true of other spices and foods as well which are not highly processed, but you get the point.

**Joel Fuhrman's** nutrient density scale is an **"aggregate nutrient density index"**. It was formed by combining weighted ORAC values (oxygen radical absorbance capacity) (a measure of the antioxidant activity of foods) with very specific plant-sourced anti-cancer compounds and with vitamins and minerals, while leaving out essential fatty acids, essential amino acids, and essential vitamins and minerals such as vitamin D2 and vitamin D3, vitamin K2, biotin, iodine, sodium, chloride, non-plant-source sulfur, boron, molybdenum, and chromium. However, the strict scientific definition of "nutrients" is: vitamins and minerals, essential fatty acids, and essential amino acids. Antioxidants are not included in the strict definition. Also, Fuhrman's list is clearly biased towards antioxidants and anti-cancerous plant foods. **Mathieu Lalonde**, on the other hand, focused on vitamins and minerals only, for his nutrient density scale. He left out sodium, chloride, chromium, iodide, molybdenum, nickel, cobalt, sulfur, lycopene, lutein, zeaxanthin, cholesterol, non essential fatty acids, lipid total, ash, protein, carbohydrates, and total sugar. He also subtracted water and fiber from all foods to obtain his values. This last subtraction is a problem in my opinion, being that fiber contains nutrients, and being that many antioxidants are actually bound with fiber (which is why making smoothies with fruits and veggies is generally better for you than juicing the fruits and veggies).

Lalonde also does not consider fiber as essential. His work was done around late 2012/early 2013, towards the beginning of the explosion of research on the microbiome. The Human Microbiome Project hadn't mapped the human microbiome until June of 2012 and hadn't reached phase two of their project until 2014. Had Lalonde done his work today, he might have reconsidered fiber as essential, being that there are more bacteria in your gut than there are cells in your body, and being that these bacteria primarily prefer fiber as their food source, from which they synthesize vitamins and from which they create postbiotics. Postbiotics allow for better absorption of minerals. The old adage or water cooler talk was that fiber blocked the absorption of vitamins and minerals, so you shouldn't take your multivitamin with anything high in fiber. But, with the knowledge we have of the microbiome now, that information isn't really very relevant anymore. Subtracting fiber also biases towards animal foods, and Lalonde is a paleo guy. Whereas plant material is very high in fiber, animal food is very low in fiber and mainly made out of protein and/or fat. Shouldn't we therefore subtract the protein from animal foods to put them on the same level as plant foods, then do our calculations? It gets complicated; it gets confusing. Lalonde says he "left out" protein, so I guess that's similar to subtracting it, but not quite the same maybe, since the subtraction of fiber is in his mathematical formula and the subtraction of protein is not.

Another difference that sets my nutrient density scale apart from Lalonde's and Fuhrman's, is that I don't combine nutrients together with each other in determining which foods are overall the most nutrient dense for a wide range of nutrients. Nor do I combine single foods and group them into overarching categories, as Lalonde does, in order to give an interpretation of which categories of foods are the most nutrient dense. I focus on each nutrient and find the specific foods that are highest in that single nutrient. For instance, I list a specific food like nettles, while Lalonde puts specific foods into groups, such as putting liver in the category of Organ meats and Oils, or garlic in the category of Herbs and Spices, or pumpkin seeds in the category of Nuts and Seeds, and so on. Of course, one could use my list of specific foods and then put them into categories and see which categories come out on top, and that is what he did, but I prefer just knowing which specific foods are high in which nutrients, not what categories are overall the most nutrient dense categories. Error and bias can come into play too when categorizing a single food. Should I put ground, dried sumac in Herbs and Spices or in Fruits? Should I put seaweed in Seafood or Vegetables? Technically speaking, seaweed is not a vegetable, but does Lalonde know that? What if he put mushrooms in the category of Vegetables also, when mushrooms are not vegetables either? You would have to make a category for mushrooms all by themselves, since they are their own kingdom in biological classification. These categorical terms are more colloquial than they are botanical and biological. Anyhow, here's exactly how Lalonde calculated his foods and how I calculated mine.

### Mathieu Lalonde's mathematical formula:

$$\textbf{Nutrient Density} = \frac{(\sum \text{Essential Nutrients Per Serving}) - \text{Sodium}}{[100 - (\text{grams of water} + \text{grams of fiber})]}$$

(Caloric Weight)

### Collin Gow, C.N.C.'s mathematical formula:

$$\textbf{Nutrient Density} = \frac{(\sum \text{Essential Nutrient Per 100g})}{[100 - (\text{grams of water})]}$$

Top 10 whole foods rich in **Calcium**, water subtracted

1. Stinging Nettles, blanched (Northern Plains Indians) 39.01mg/g
2. Rhubarb, frozen, uncooked 29.89mg/g
3. Nopales, raw 27.89mg/g
4. Mustard spinach (tendergreen), raw 26.92mg/g
5. Amaranth leaves, raw 25.87mg/g
6. Spices, basil, dried 24.99mg/g
7. Lambs quarters, raw (Northern Plains Indians) 24.78mg/g
8. Spices, savory, ground 23.43mg/g
9. Collards, raw 22.35mg/g
10. Spices, marjoram, dried 21.55mg/g

Top 10 whole foods rich in **Iron**, water subtracted

1. Beef, variety meats and by-products, spleen, raw 1.95mg/g Other spleens
2. Spices, thyme, dried 1.34mg/g
3. Mushrooms, morel, raw 1.17mg/g
4. Duck, domesticated, liver, raw 1.08mg/g Other livers
5. Spices, basil, dried 1.00mg/g
6. Spearmint, dried .99mg/g
7. Whale, beluga, meat, dried (Alaska Native) .93mg/g
8. Spices, marjoram, dried .90mg/g
9. Pork, fresh, variety meats and by-products, lungs, cooked, braised .82mg/g
10. Seaweed, Canadian Cultivated EMI-TSUNOMATA, dry .77mg/g

Top 10 whole foods rich in **Magnesium**, water subtracted

1. Beverages, coffee, brewed, espresso, restaurant-prepared 36.36mg/g
2. Dock, raw 14.71mg/g (Docks and sorrels, genus Rumex, leaves edible)
3. Mollusks, snail, raw 12.02mg/g
4. Chard, swiss, cooked, boiled, drained, without salt 11.56mg/g
5. Epazote, raw 11.21mg/g
6. Lambsquarters, steamed (Northern Plains Indians) 10.95mg/g
7. Purslane, cooked, boiled, drained, without salt 10.34mg/g
8. Spinach, cooked, boiled, drained, without salt 9.90mg/g
9. Swamp cabbage, (skunk cabbage), raw 9.43mg/g
10. Nopales, raw 8.84mg/g

Top 10 whole foods rich in **Potassium**, water subtracted

1. Bamboo shoots, cooked, boiled, drained, without salt 130.64mg/g
2. Butterbur, (fuki), raw 119.09mg/g
3. Cabbage, japanese style, fresh, pickled 99.19mg/g and Chinese and others
4. Lambsquarters, raw (Northern Plains Indians) 85.99mg/g
5. Beet greens, cooked, boiled, drained, without salt 83.62mg/g
6. Chrysanthemum, garland, cooked, boiled, drained, without salt 75.77mg/g
7. Amaranth leaves, cooked, boiled, drained, without salt 75.32mg/g
8. Chard, swiss, cooked, boiled, drained, without salt 74.69mg/g
9. Taro shoots, cooked, without salt 73.19mg/g

10. Purslane, raw 69.19mg/g

Top 10 whole foods rich in **Zinc**, water subtracted

1. Mollusks, oyster, eastern, canned 6.12mg/g multiple
2. Veal, variety meats and by-products, liver, raw .41mg/g
3. Crustaceans, crab, alaska king, cooked, moist heat .34mg/g
4. Beef, ribeye petite roast, boneless, separable lean only, trimmed to 0" fat, select, cooked, roasted .31mg/g
5. Lamb, Australian, imported, fresh, foreshank, separable lean only, trimmed to 1/8" fat, cooked, braised.24mg/g
6. Chicken, heart, all classes, cooked, simmered.21mg/g
7. Game meat, bear, cooked, simmered .22mg/g
8. Game meat, bison, chuck, shoulder clod, separable lean only, cooked, braised .22mg/g
9. Emu, oyster, raw .22mg/g
10. Crustaceans, spiny lobster, mixed species, cooked, moist heat .22mg/g

I must give another **caveat** here. In my water subtracted lists in this article, I did leave out some foods that were so similar that it made no sense to leave them in. For instance, instead of including both "Beef, ribeye, petite roast" and "Beef, ribeye, filet", I simply got rid of the filet, since the petite roast was higher on the list, and there's no use populating the whole list with different versions or cuts or cooking techniques of nearly the same food, "Beef". Another example is "Lamb, Australian, imported, fresh, foreshank" and "Lamb, domestic, foreshank". I left off the second lamb here because it was lower on the list than the first and a nearly identical food. If I hadn't left any foods out, this would be the real list for Zinc (two foods—emu testicle and lobster—wouldn't have made the top 10):

Top 10 whole foods rich in **Zinc**, water subtracted

1. Mollusks, oyster, eastern, canned 6.12mg/g multiple
2. Veal, variety meats and by-products, liver, raw .41mg/g
3. Crustaceans, crab, alaska king, cooked, moist heat .34mg/g
4. Beef, ribeye petite roast, boneless, separable lean only, trimmed to 0" fat, select, cooked, roasted .31mg/g
5. Beef, ribeye filet, boneless, separable lean only, trimmed to 0" fat, select, cooked, grilled . 29mg/g
6. Lamb, Australian, imported, fresh, foreshank, separable lean only, trimmed to 1/8" fat, cooked, braised.24mg/g
7. Lamb, domestic, foreshank, separable lean only, trimmed to 1/4" fat, choice, cooked, braised . 23mg/g
8. Chicken, heart, all classes, cooked, simmered.21mg/g
9. Game meat, bear, cooked, simmered .22mg/g
10. Game meat, bison, chuck, shoulder clod, separable lean only, cooked, braised .22mg/g

When I got to this point in my water subtracted calculations, I became very tired of calculating and configuring these lists, since I had already spent hours researching the subject and spent many hours making 4 other versions of these lists with different methods of calculation prior to arriving at my water subtracted method. Therefore, I leave it to you, my reader, to calculate the rest of the nutrients in the method I've shared. **Here is the current link to the USDA's database:**

https://fdc.nal.usda.gov/. However, I won't just totally leave you hanging, knowing only 5 nutrients in foods. **Below are the simplest lists of the nutrient data, just accounting for how many mg of a nutrient are in 100g of real food and doing nothing else—no subtracting water, no removing similar foods, no calculating involved whatsoever.** As you can see, the lists are dominated by slight variations of the same foods. However, this information is better than nothing. You can see why organ meats have been hailed as the most nutrient dense foods on the planet, since they generally dominate the lists:

Vitamin A
1. Braised moose liver
2. Raw walrus liver
3. Raw broccoli leaves
4. Simmered turkey liver
5. Raw turkey liver
6. Braised veal liver
7. Raw duck liver
8. Raw veal liver
9. Simmered turkey giblets
10. Braised beef liver

Vitamin Bp (Choline)
1. Raw egg yolk
2. Simmered beef kidneys
3. Simmered beef brain
4. Black and red caviar
5. Simmered pork chitterlings (intestine)
6. Braised beef liver
7. Pan-fried beef liver
8. Pain-fried veal liver
9. Braised veal liver
10. Raw fish roe (mixed species)

Vitamin B1 (Thiamin)
1. Flax seeds
2. Sesame butter
3. Dried sunflower seeds
4. Cilantro
5. Dried pine nuts
6. Raw macadamia nuts
7. Dried Safflower seed kernels
8. Multiple kinds of pork
9. Dried pilinuts
10. More pork

Vitamin B2 (Riboflavin)
1. Pan-fried lamb liver
2. Braised moose liver

3. Braised lamb liver
4. Raw lamb liver
5. Braised beef liver
6. Pan-fried beef liver
7. Pan-fried veal liver
8. Raw pork liver
9. Simmered beef kidneys
10. Braised veal liver

Vitamin B3 (Niacin)

1. Smoked sockeye salmon with skin on
2. Anchovies
3. Tuna
4. Braised beef liver
5. Pan-fried beef liver
6. Whole dried sisymbrium seeds (hedge mustard seeds)
7. Pan-fried lamb liver
8. Raw lamb liver
9. Raw Spanish peanuts
10. Raw skipjack tuna

Folate

1. Raw duck liver
2. Raw goose liver
3. Simmered turkey liver
4. Raw turkey liver
5. Raw chicken liver
6. Simmered chicken liver
7. Pan-fried chicken liver
8. Simmered chicken giblets
9. Pan-fried lamb liver
10. Raw capon giblets (rooster giblets)

Vitamin B5 (Pantethenic Acid)

1. Pan-fried chicken liver
2. Raw beef liver
3. Braised beef liver
4. Pan-fried veal liver
5. Toasted sunflower seed kernels
6. Dry roasted sunflower seed kernels
7. Sunflower seed butter
8. Pan-fried beef liver
9. Simmered chicken liver
10. Raw pork liver

Vitamin B6 (pyridoxine)

1. Raw pistachio nuts

2. Raw turkey liver
3. Dried sunflower seeds
4. Dry roasted pistachio nuts
5. Raw garlic
6. Raw horseradish tree leafy tips
7. Dried safflower seed kernels
8. Raw beef liver
9. Simmered turkey liver
10. Dry heat cooked yellowfin tuna

Vitamin b12 (cobalamin)

1. Canned, drained clams
2. Moist heat cooked clams, mixed species
3. Raw lamb liver
4. Pan-fried lamb liver
5. Braised veal liver
6. Pan-fried beef liver
7. Braise lamb kidneys
8. Braised lamb liver
9. Pan-fried veal liver
10. Braised moose liver

Vitamin C

1. Raw acerola cherries
2. Raw acerola juice
3. Wild rose hips
4. Raw green hot chili peppers
5. Raw common guavas
6. Chopped young willow leaves
7. Raw yellow sweet peppers
8. Raw European black currants
9. Sauteed green sweet peppers
10. Boiled, drained red sweet peppers

Vitamin D

1. Raw Atlantic herring
2. Canned sockeye salmon with bones
3. Pickled Atlantic herring
4. Canned pink salmon with bones and liquid
5. Boiled, canned steelhead trout
6. Raw Greenland halibut
7. Raw wild catfish
8. Canned pink salmon drained with bone
9. Raw Atlantic Mackerel
10. Raw wild eastern oysters

Vitamin E (alpha tocopherol)

1. Dried sunflower seeds
2. Almonds
3. Dry roasted sunflower seeds
4. Dry roasted almonds
5. Blanched almonds
6. Blanched hazelnuts
7. Dry roasted hazelnuts
8. Hazelnuts
9. Roasted pinon nuts
10. Dried Pine nuts

Vitamin E (Gamma Tocopherol)

1. Pecans
2. Dry roasted pecans
3. Raw pistachio nuts
4. Dry roasted pistachio nuts
5. English walnuts
6. Flaxseeds
7. Dried pumpkin and squash kernels
8. Yellow mustard seed
9. Dried pine nuts
10. Poppy seeds

Vitamin K

1. Raw parsley
2. Raw amaranth leaves
3. Frozen boiled kale, drained
4. Raw swiss chard
5. Kale boiled, drained
6. Raw kale
7. Raw dandelion greens
8. Frozen collards boiled, drained
9. Dandelion greens boiled, drained
10. Raw garden cress

Calcium

1. Celery seed
2. Sisymbrium seeds, dried (hedg mustard)
3. Dill seed
4. Poppy seeds
5. Parmesan cheese
6. Parmesan cheese shredded
7. Fennel seeds
8. Hard parmesan cheese
9. Grated parmesan cheese
10. Romano cheese

Iron

1. Cumin seeds
2. Celery seed
3. Raw lamb spleen
4. Braised beef spleen
5. Braised lamb spleen
6. Anise seeds
7. Fenugreek seeds
8. Raw duck liver
9. Raw goose liver
10. Black pepper

Magnesium

1. Dried pumpkin and squash seed kernels
2. Roasted pumpkin and squash seed kernels
3. Dried watermelon seed kernels
4. Celery seeds
5. Flaxseeds
6. Fennel seeds
7. Brazilnuts
8. Sunflower seed butter
9. Cumin seed
10. Sesame seed butter

Potassium

1. Sisymbrium seeds (hedge mustard)
2. Breadnut tree seeds
3. Palm hearts raw
4. Cumin seeds
5. Fennel seeds
6. Roasted soybeans
7. Molasses
8. Anise seeds
9. Gjetost cheese
10. Celery seed

Zinc

1. Moist heat cooked wild eastern oysters
2. Canned eastern oysters
3. Raw wild eastern oysters
4. Dry heat cooked wild eastern oysters
5. Dry heat cooked farmed eastern oysters
6. Raw farmed eastern oysters
7. Moist heat cooked Pacific oysters
8. Raw Pacific oysters
9. Raw veal liver
10. Pan-fried veal liver

Copper
1. Pan-fried veal liver
2. Braised veal liver
3. Pan-fried beef liver
4. Braised beef liver
5. Raw veal liver
6. Pan-fried lamb liver
7. Raw beef liver
8. Moist heat cooked wild eastern oysters
9. Raw goose liver
10. Braised lamb liver

Manganese
1. Blanched hazelnuts
2. Dried pine nuts
3. Celery seed
4. Moist heat cooked blue mussels
5. Poppy seeds
6. Raw fireweed leaves
7. Dried butternuts
8. Fennel seeds
9. Hazelnuts
10. Dry roasted hazelnuts

Selenium
1. Unblanched dried brazilnuts
2. Sea lion liver
3. Braised pork kidneys
4. Braised lamb kidneys
5. Raw pork kidneys
6. Simmered beef kidneys
7. Moist heat cooked Pacific oysters
8. Raw turkey giblets
9. Raw beef kidneys
10. Yellow mustard seeds

Fluoride
1. Seedless raisins
2. Canned blue crab
3. White wine, table
4. Canned shrimp, mixed species
5. Grape juice, unsweetened canned or bottled
6. Red wine, table
7. Merlot table red wine
8. Grape soda
9. Tonic water
10. Municipal tap water

# Alkaline/Neutral/Acidic Foods Simplified

Collin Gow, C.N.C. (2022)

## Alkaline

- Fruit (except tart/sour fruits*)
- Vegetables
- Herbs and Spices (except tart/sour ones*)

## Neutral

- Millet
- Fats, Oils, Milk (Remer et al., 1995)

## Acidic

- Everything Else

***I do not completely subscribe to the alkaline/acid-ash hypothesis.**

# High Anti-oxidant/ Anti-inflammatory Foods

Collin Gow, C.N.C. (2022)

Raw, organic, colorful, whole plant foods, beverages, and/or essential oils such as:

- **Herbs and Spices**, especially sumac, cloves, allspice, mint, cinnamon, oregano, Mexican oregano, thyme, sage, celery seeds, and rosemary
- **Vegetables**, especially parsley, beets, broccoli, eggplant, Brussels sprouts, cabbage, asparagus, red peppers, and hot peppers
- **Leaves**, especially pomegranate leaves, olive leaves, curry leaves, and African baobab leaves
- **Fruits**, especially amla, bilberries, blackberries, red currants, raspberries, blueberries, citrus, pineapple, and papaya
- **"Superfoods"**, especially amla, acai, maqui, goldenberries, etc.
- **Nuts and Seeds**, especially walnuts, pecans, brazil nuts, and black sesame seeds
- **Dark Chocolate, 90% Cacao or higher** (doesn't need to be raw)
- **Espresso and Coffee** (shouldn't be raw)
- **Seaweeds**, especially brown seaweeds
- **Dog Rose and Dog Rose Hips**
- **Black rice and Rice Koji miso**
- **Tea,** especially hibiscus, matcha, oolong, sencha, and pu-erh
- **Black Soybeans**

References:


1. Carlsen MH, Halvorsen BL, Holte K, Bøhn SK, Dragland S, Sampson L, Willey C, Senoo H, Umezono Y, Sanada C, Barikmo I, Berhe N, Willett WC, Phillips KM, Jacobs DR Jr, Blomhoff R. The total antioxidant content of more than 3100 foods, beverages, spices, herbs and supplements used worldwide. Nutr J. 2010 Jan 22;9:3. doi: 10.1186/1475-2891-9-3. PMID: 20096093; PMCID: PMC2841576.
2. Yashin A, Yashin Y, Xia X, Nemzer B. Antioxidant Activity of Spices and Their Impact on Human Health: A Review. Antioxidants (Basel). 2017 Sep 15;6(3):70. doi: 10.3390/antiox6030070. PMID: 28914764; PMCID: PMC5618098.
3. Xu DP, Li Y, Meng X, Zhou T, Zhou Y, Zheng J, Zhang JJ, Li HB. Natural Antioxidants in Foods and Medicinal Plants: Extraction, Assessment and Resources. Int J Mol Sci. 2017 Jan 5;18(1):96. doi: 10.3390/ijms18010096. PMID: 28067795; PMCID: PMC5297730.
4. Waisundara V, Yian Hoon L. A comparative study on the antioxidant activity of commonly used South asian herbs. J Tradit Complement Med. 2013 Oct;3(4):263-7. doi: 10.4103/2225-4110.119725. PMID: 24716187; PMCID: PMC3924994.

5. Pellegrini N, Serafini M, Colombi B, Del Rio D, Salvatore S, Bianchi M, Brighenti F. Total antioxidant capacity of plant foods, beverages and oils consumed in Italy assessed by three different in vitro assays. J Nutr. 2003 Sep;133(9):2812-9. doi: 10.1093/jn/133.9.2812. PMID: 12949370.
6. Tsubota-Utsugi M, Watanabe J, Takebayashi J, Oki T, Tsubono Y, Ohkubo T. The Major Source of Antioxidants Intake From Typical Diet Among Rural Farmers in North-eastern Japan in the 1990s. J Epidemiol. 2021 Feb 5;31(2):101-108. doi: 10.2188/jea.JE20190237. Epub 2020 Jan 25. PMID: 31983720; PMCID: PMC7813768.
7. Pisoschi AM, Pop A, Cimpeanu C, Predoi G. Antioxidant Capacity Determination in Plants and Plant-Derived Products: A Review. Oxid Med Cell Longev. 2016;2016:9130976. doi: 10.1155/2016/9130976. Epub 2016 Dec 4. PMID: 28044094; PMCID: PMC5164913.
8. Song W, Derito CM, Liu MK, He X, Dong M, Liu RH. Cellular antioxidant activity of common vegetables. J Agric Food Chem. 2010 Jun 9;58(11):6621-9. doi: 10.1021/jf9035832. PMID: 20462192.
9. Schauss AG, Wu X, Prior RL, Ou B, Huang D, Owens J, Agarwal A, Jensen GS, Hart AN, Shanbrom E. Antioxidant capacity and other bioactivities of the freeze-dried Amazonian palm berry, Euterpe oleraceae mart. (acai). J Agric Food Chem. 2006 Nov 1;54(22):8604-10. doi: 10.1021/jf0609779. PMID: 17061840.
10. Turner-McGrievy GM, Wirth MD, Shivappa N, Wingard EE, Fayad R, Wilcox S, Frongillo EA, Hébert JR. Randomization to plant-based dietary approaches leads to larger short-term improvements in Dietary Inflammatory Index scores and macronutrient intake compared with diets that contain meat. Nutr Res. 2015 Feb;35(2):97-106. doi: 10.1016/j.nutres.2014.11.007. Epub 2014 Dec 3. PMID: 25532675.

# Blood Type Foods & Personality

Collin Gow, C.N.C. (2022)

## Type O

A **pre-agriculture, hunter-gatherer, wild, paleo type diet**. Type O's require more protein, iron, iodine, calcium, and vitamin K1. Limit grains, legumes, high glycemic carbs, and dairy. The most ancient blood type. The most common blood type in America. Roughly 40% of the population. Generally suffer from anemia, thyroid issues, Crohn's, and colitis. Hypervigilant/hyperactive immune system that fights everything that comes along. A driven, confident, resilient, intuitive, intense, reactive, strong, daring, risk-taker, with endurance, optimism, passion, and self-reliance. Can be self-centered at times.

## Type A

**Plant-based diet**. Thrives on fruits, veggies, and carbohydrate foods. Sensitive gut. Limit animal proteins, tomatoes, and dairy. The second blood type to develop on the evolutionary timeline. Generally suffer from low stomach acid, which may cause acid reflux, and at a higher risk for stomach cancer, breast cancer, and ear infections. Immune system can be too tolerant of pathogens and not fight them often enough. Law abiding, cooperative, sedentary, patient, loyal, tactful, uptight, stubborn, clever, anxious.

## Type B

A **balanced, flexible, various, omnivorous diet**. The 3rd blood type to come along. Has a strong immune system and a tolerant digestive tract. Can consume dairy. May be more prone to MS, Lupus, or CFS. Have a harmonious personality and are empathetic and decisive, yet sometimes selfish and uncooperative. Dislike authority.

## Type AB

A **mixed diet**. Less than 5% of the population. A merging of A and B blood type/diet. The most modern blood type. Immune system can be sluggish and overly tolerant of pathogens, not doing much to fight them. May be more prone to gastric and pancreatic cancer. May be somewhat flaky, indecisive, forgetful, and hard to read, yet are not fussy about details and are spiritual. May have a dual personality and can be captivating, charismatic, diplomatic, and popular, yet loyal to no one group.

# Pathogens

# Berberine: Pathogen Profile

Collin Gow, C.N.C.

3/12/2022

**Berberine** may inhibit/kill the following Harmful Bacteria including:

- Chlamydia species including:
- Chlamydia pneumoniae
- Chlamydia trachomatis
- Cornybacterium diptheria
- Enterococcus species
- Escherichia coli
- Helicobacter pylori
- Mycobacterium tuberculosis
- Neisseria gonorrhoeae
- Neisseria memingitidis
- Porphyromonas gingivalis
- Pseudomonas species
- Salmonella typhi
- Shigella dysenteriae
- Staphylococcus species including:
- Methicillin Resistant Staphylococcus aureus (MRSA)
- Streptomyces species
- Treponema pallidum
- Vibrio cholerae

Berberine may destroy some forms of Detrimental Fungi:

- Candida albicans
- Candida krusei

Berberine may inhibit/kill these Deleterious Parasites:

- Entamoeba histolytica in the Gastrointestinal Tract
- Giardia lamblia that causes Giardiasis
- Trichomonas vaginalis

Berberine may inhibit some types of Viruses:

- Herpes Simplex Virus Type 1
- Herpes Simplex Virus Type 2
- Influenza Viruses

Berberine may stimulate the Immune System:
Berberine may benefit Macrophages and improve the activity of the Spleen
Berberine may reduce Inflammation

(Obtained from In-Tele-Health's Hyperhealth Pro 11, 2012)

# Garlic: Pathogen Profile

Collin Gow, C.N.C.

3/9/2022

**Garlic** may stimulate Immunity:

- May stimulate Lymphocytes to destroy Antigens
- May activate Macrophages to destroy Antigens
- May improve the ability of NK Lymphocytes to destroy Antigens
- May potentiate the Lymphokine-activated killer cell action of T-Lymphocytes

Garlic may kill/inhibit/suppress the following Bacteria:

- Bacillus anthracis
- Bacillus cereus
- Bacillus subtilis
- Clostridium perfringens
- Escherichia coli
- Helicobacter pylori
- Klebsiella pneumoniae
- Mycobacterium smegmatis
- Proteus vulgaris
- Salmonella species:
- Salmonella enteritidis
- Salmonella typhi
- Porphyromonas gingivalis
- Shigella Bacteria
- Staphylococcus epidermidis.
- Staphylococcus aureus.
- Streptococcus Bacteria:
- Streptococcus mutans
- Streptococcus pneumoniae
- Streptomyces griseus
- Xanthomonas maltophilia

Garlic may kill/suppress many types of Harmful Fungi:

- Aspergillus flavus
- Aspergillus fumigatus
- Aspergillus niger
- Candida albicans
- Cryptococcus neoformans
- Dermatophytes
- Garlic may reduce the toxicity of Aflatoxin

Garlic may counteract Detrimental Parasites:

- Cryptosporidium parvum
- Entamoeba histolytica
- Giardia lamblia that causes Giardiasis
- Plasmodium that causes Malaria

Garlic may help in the Destruction of some kinds of Viruses:

- May help to restore NK Lymphocyte activity and improve the Helper/Suppressor T-cell ratio in AIDS patients
- May protect against the Viruses that cause the Common Cold and may improve the symptoms of the Common Cold
- Cytomegalovirus (CMV)
- Symptoms of Influenza
- Inhibit Papillomas
- Rotavirus

(Obtained from In-Tele-Health's Hyperhealth Pro 11, 2012)

# Grapefruit Seed Extract: Pathogen Profile

Collin Gow, C.N.C.

7/5/2021

**Grapefruit Seed extract** may kill or suppress many (over 900) Detrimental Microorganisms:

Grapefruit Seed extract may kill or inhibit the growth of the following Deleterious Bacteria including:

- Bacillus anthracis (possibly)
- Bacillus subtilis
- Bacillus cereus
- Borrelia burgdorferi (causes Lyme disease)
- Brucella abortus
- Escherichia coli
- Campylobacter jejuni
- Chlamydia trachomatis
- Clostridium botulinum
- Clostridium tetani
- Corynebacterium diphtheriae
- Haemophilus influenzae
- Helicobacter pylori
- Klebsiella pneumoniae
- Legionella pneumoniae
- Listeria monocytogenes
- Moraxella catarrhalis
- Mycobacterium smegmatis
- Mycobacterium tuberculosis
- Mycoplasma species
- Pasteurella septica
- Propionibacterium acnes
- Proteus mirabilis
- Proteus vulgaris
- Pseudomonas aeruginosa
- Pseudomonas cepacia
- Salmonella enteridis
- Salmonella choleraesuis
- Salmonella enteritidis
- Salmonella paratyphi A
- Salmonella typhi
- Serratia marcescens
- Shigella dysenteriae
- Shigella flexneri
- Shigella sonnei

- Staphylococcus aureus
- Streptococcus faecalis
- Streptococcus pneumoniae
- Streptococcus pyogenes
- Streptococcus viridans
- Vancomycin-Resistant Enterococcus (VRE)
- Vibrio cholerae

Grapefruit Seed extract may inhibit some species of Detrimental Fungi, Detrimental Molds and Detrimental Yeasts including:

- Aspergillus
- Candida albicans (regarded by some as the best treatment against Candida albicans infection)
- Trichophyton mentagrophytes

Grapefruit Seed extract may inhibit these Pernicious Parasites:

- Blastocystis hominis
- Entamoeba histolytica (responsible for Amebiasis)
- Giardia lamblia (cause of Giardiasis)

Grapefruit Seed extract may inhibit some types of Viruses:

- HIV virus (possibly)
- Bacteriophage T1
- Bacteriophage T7
- Coronaviruses
- Herpes Simplex Virus Type 1
- Herpes Zoster Virus
- Influenza
- Measles Virus

Grapefruit Seed extract is claimed to kill all types of Intestinal Parasites

(Obtained from In-Tele-Health's Hyperhealth Pro 11, 2012)

# Oregano Oil: Pathogen Profile

Collin Gow, C.N.C.

5/16/2021

**Oregano Oil** may alleviate many inhibit/kill a range of Detrimental Bacteria and Viruses

Oregano Oil may inhibit (and may sometimes kill) many types of Bad Bacteria including:

- Bacillus cereus
- Escherichia coli
- Klebsiella pneumoniae
- Mycobacterium paratuberculosis
- Pseudomonas aeruginosa
- Salmonella
- Staphylococcus:
- Staphylococcus aureus
- Streptococcus:
- Streptococcus pneumoniae

Oregano Oil may alleviate or accelerate the recovery from the Common Cold

Oregano Oil may inhibit (and may sometimes kill) several types of Toxic Fungi and Harmful Yeasts:

- Aspergillus flavus
- Aspergillus parasiticus
- Candida albicans

Oregano Oil may fight several Detrimental Parasites including:

- Blastocystis hominis
- Endolimax nana
- Entamoeba hartmanni
- Giardia lamblia (the cause of Giardiasis)

Oregano Oil (600 mg per day) may help to kill Intestinal Parasites

Oregano Oil may increase Lymph flow

Oregano Oil is antiviral (it disintegrates the outer membrane of some Viruses) including:

- Herpes Simplex Virus Type 1
- Newcastle Disease Virus

(Obtained from In-Tele-Health's Hyperhealth Pro 11, 2012)

# Silver: Pathogen Profile

Collin Gow, C.N.C.

3/12/2022

**Silver** may kill many Harmful Bacteria including:

- Actinomyces species
- Bacillus anthracis (the cause of Anthrax)
- Bacillus cereus
- Bacillus subtilis
- Bordetella pertussis
- Brucella species
- Chlamydia psittaci
- Chlamydia trachomatis
- Enterococcus faecalis
- Escherichia coli
- Mycoplasma species
- Neisseria gonorrhoeae (the Detrimental Bacteria that causes Gonhorrhea)
- Pseudomonas aeruginosa
- Staphylococcus aureus
- Streptococcus pneumoniae
- Vibrio cholerae (the cause of Cholera)

Silver may be a potent exterminator of some types of Detrimental Fungi:

- Aspergillus niger
- Candida albicans
- Cryptococcus neoformans

Silver may kill some Harmful Parasites including:

- Entamoeba histolytica
- Paramecium

Silver may help to kill Intestinal Parasites

Silver may counteract some Viruses:

- HIV
- Cytomegalovirus (CMV)
- Epstein-Barr Virus (EBV)
- Herpes Simplex Virus Type 1
- Herpes Simplex Virus Type 2
- Herpes Zoster Virus (the cause of Shingles)
- Influenza Viruses

(Obtained from In-Tele-Health's Hyperhealth Pro 11, 2012)

# Education Curriculum

**“Nature is health and health is nature.”**

**“Be a Naturevore. Eat nature.”**

# Collin Gow, C.N.C.'s

# Wholistic, Scientific, Individualized, Nature-Inspired, Whole Health, Nutrition, and Wellness Education Curriculum

## (Ages 5–18)

**“To become whole is to heal.”**

**“Our aim is not self-actualization, it is self-naturalization.”**

# My Skills, Knowledge, Credentials, and Experience

- 13 years of experience as a certified nutritional consultant

- Published author of 5 books

- Over 100 lectures on YouTube and I have appeared on radio, TV, and in print

- I'm a father and have been teaching my son health, nutrition, healthy foods, Spanish, healthy cooking, shopping for health food, nature spirituality, gardening, physical fitness, ethics, morals, and foraging for the past 6 years and homeschooling him for the past year

- I have attended kids gardening and farming classes

- I have attended kids cooking workshops

- I grow 40 plants myself and forage wild edible foods

- Kids love me. I am able to become a kid when I'm around them and play with them while teaching them valuable life skills

# Syllabus

**Title:** *Collin Gow, C.N.C.'s Wholistic, Scientific, Individualized, Nature-Inspired, Whole Health, Nutrition, and Wellness Education Curriculum (Ages 5–18)*

**No. of Credits:** .5

**Department:** Nutrition

**Pre-requisites:** none

**Course Teacher:** you

**Learning Hours:** 22.5 Hours—Lecture (7.5 hours); Activity (15 hours)

**Course Description:** a comprehensive, wholistic, scientific, individualized, nature-inspired, integrative, exciting, engaging, varied, creative, and challenging health, nutrition, and wellness course written by a certified nutritional consultant with 13 years of experience. There would be different instructions within it for ages 5–11 and ages 12–18. This course would include guidelines for lectures as well as links to video lectures done by Collin, plus hands-on, fun, and educational lessons, worksheets, activities, and field trips to aid students on their journeys towards whole health, wellness, and self-naturalization. The course would offer opportunities for self-directed learning and group learning and it would interweave not only nutrition, but healthy lifestyle behaviors, activities, and attitudes as well. It not only focuses on physical health, rather, it assists the child or adolescent in becoming a whole person. To become whole is to heal. (This is an outline of a course. It may be used as part of a child or adolescent's homeschool studies. If you or your school would like to purchase or license the full, in-depth course, contact collingowcnc@gmail.com)

**Course Objectives:** know what it means to be healthy, why it's important, and how to get healthy. Know what foods are healthy, know what nutrients are high in common foods, know how to put together and be able to cook a healthy meal, know what plants are edible and healthy in the wild, know what organs and tissues in the body do what, know what foods resemble what organs and tissues and are therfore good for those organs and tissues, know how to shop for healthy foods, know how to grow healthy foods, know where food comes from, know different foods around the world and how to say them in a different language, know healthy ways to exercise, reconnect with the earth, and get outside into nature. Learn how to bring nature to you, how to take care of the earth, and how and when to celebrate nature.

**Course Content:** this course covers the subjects of health (mind, body, emotional, behavioral, and spiritual), nutrition, healthy foods (in America and around the world), healthy ways to create a meal and cook a meal (with recipes), healthy shopping, nature wisdom, natural movement (physical exercise), lifestyle factors, how to garden/how to grow food, foraging/plant identification, where food comes from, anatomy/physiology functions, foods for particular parts of the body, environmentalism/taking care of the earth (where health comes from), and celebrating nature.

**Course Learning Outcomes:** I will learn what it means to be healthy, why it's important to be healthy, and how to be healthy. I will become better equipped to discern between what is healthy and what is not. I will be able to take my health into my own hands. I will gain skills to enact healthy behaviors, actions, and attitudes. I will become more connected with nature and my own body, mind, emotions, and spirit. I will learn survival skills. I will become whole. I will become healthy. I will become a natural human animal. I will learn that nature is where health comes from. I will become self-naturalized.

**Course Assessment Methods:** Portfolio, ipsative methods, quizzes, projects, student interview, group discussions/activities/participation, and presentations

**Materials Required:** old clothing or clothing scraps, scissors, construction paper, card-stock, plastic foods and plastic plates (optional), real foods, kitchen supplies, proximity to a park, field, or nature-preserve, pen or pencil, markers or crayons or paints and paint brush, white paper, Leap Frog Academy device and Captain Plasma game (optional), Farming board game (optional), two planter pots, soil, small shovel, two different packets of seeds, access to a grocery store or health food store, clean water, disposable gloves, trash bags, birdseed, squirrel baffle, chain or rope, and upcycled bird feeder materials such as citrus rinds and string, or paper towel rolls, sunflower butter, and string, or plant milk carton and string, or two liter bottles, dowel rods, and shoe-laces or string or chain.

**Grading Guidelines:** Portfolio: 50%, Ipsative: 20%, Quizzes: 10%, Projects/Homework: 10%, Student Interview: 5%, Group Discussions/Activities/Participation: 2.5%, Presentations: 2.5%

# Lessons

# Lesson 1

## Lecture:

- What is health?
- What does it mean to be healthy?
- Why is it important to be healthy?
- Why is it important to eat healthy food?
- What foods are healthy?

## Homework or Activity:

- Make a costume or t-shirt of, or dress up as, your favorite healthy food

# Lesson 2

## Lecture:

- What does a healthy meal look like?

## Activity:

- Draw 1 healthy meal based on the principles learned or create 1 healthy meal with construction paper and scissors or create 5 different healthy meals with toy foods and toy plates or make silly faces with real, healthy foods, then eat it

# Lesson 3

## <u>Lecture</u>:

- What foods are high in what nutrients?

## <u>Activity</u>:

- Create flash cards that pair nutrients and foods with each other

# Lesson 4

## Lecture:

- Anatomy and Physiology. What organs and tissues do what?

## Activity:

- Play an anatomy and physiology game, computer game, or board game to learn anatomy

# Lesson 5

## Lecture:

- What foods are good for what part of the body? (Doctrine of Signatures)

## Activity:

- Match each food with the body part it's good for

# Lesson 6

## Lecture:

- Where does food come from?

## Activity:

- Identify each food and its source

# Lesson 7

## Lecture:

- How to grow food

## Activity:

- Create a garden in pots or raised beds, or go to a community farm to learn about seeds, planting, placement, sun, soil, care, watering, etc..Or start a sprouting jar.

# Lesson 8

## <u>Lecture</u>:

- How to cook food. Healthy ways to cook food.

## <u>Activity</u>:

- Make a healthy recipe with simple ingredients and simple "cooking" techniques. Or do a fun, blind-folded taste test before-hand or in another lesson to familiarize the student with different flavors and seasonings.

# Lesson 9

## <u>Field Trip</u>:

- To a local nature preserve to take a nature walk and identify and forage native, wild, edible foods

# Lesson 10

## <u>Field Trip</u>:

- To a health food store to learn how to shop for healthy foods and what to look for on labels. Turn it into a scavenger hunt to find a list of items/words/symbols.

# Lesson 11

## <u>Lecture</u>:

- Foods around the world: Latin Countries

## <u>Activity</u>:

- Learning and pronouncing the names of healthy foods in Spanish

# Lesson 12

## Lecture:

- Learning healthy lifestyle behaviors, activities, and attitudes such as natural movement (exercise), reading, journaling, doing what you love, creating, meditating, engaging in a community, getting outside, breathing, hydrating, sleeping/waking, and practicing mindfulness, self-awareness, self-control, gratitude, acts of kindness, ethics, goal-setting, and positive balance. Generally learning mental, spiritual, emotional, and behavioral health.

## Activity:

- Answer a questionnaire on how you could engage in the healthy lifestyle factors listed or some of your favorite ways to engage in them. Or, actually carry out one of them and document what you did.

# Lesson 13

## Lecture:

- How to bring nature to you

## Activity:

- Make a bird feeder, plant a garden, gather wild flowers and put in a vase, or harvest plants from the wild and put in pots. What are some other ideas you have?

# Lesson 14

## Lecture:

- How to take care of and be a steward of the planet and why it's important

## Activity:

- Pick up trash around school or where you live

# Lesson 15

## <u>Lecture</u>:

- Natural holidays: seasons, solstices, and equinoxes. Spring Equinox, Earth Day, Summer Solstice, Fall Equinox, Winter Solstice.

## <u>Activity</u>:

- Pick a natural holiday and make an art piece, craft, or altar in honor of the correspondences (including foods) of that natural holiday

# Vaccines
# &
# COVID-19

# Post COVID-19 Vaccine Care

Collin Gow, C.N.C.
11/8/2021

It is important to know that many **side effects** have been reported by individuals after receiving COVID-19 “vaccinations”. Anyone can report their adverse reactions to the **Vaccine Adverse Events Reporting System (VAERS)** at vaers.hhs.gov. VAERS is an early warning system that monitors vaccine safety in the U.S.. It is co-managed by the **FDA** and **CDC**. As of 10/22/21, **837,595 adverse events**, **including 17,619 deaths**, have been **reported** to VAERS after COVID-19 vaccination. The following table lists some of the current adverse events that have been reported to VAERS and the number of reports:

| | |
|---|---|
| Guillain-Barre | 1537 |
| Acute Disseminated Encephalomyelitis | 108 |
| Transverse Myelitis | 280 |
| Encephalitis | 1271 |
| Convulsions/Seizures | 10618 |
| Stroke | 9952 |
| Narcolepsy, Cataplexy | 200 |
| Anaphylaxis | 37281 |
| Acute Myocardial Infarction (Heart Attack) | 2840 |
| Myocarditis/Pericarditis | 9487 |
| Autoimmune Disease | 856 |
| Other Acute Demyelinating Diseases | 204 |
| Pregnancy and birth outcomes (Miscarriages) | 2526 |
| Other Allergic Reactions | 1601 |
| Thrombocytopenia | 3456 |
| Disseminated Intravascular Coagulation | 151 |
| Venous Thromboembolism | 15287 |
| Arthritis and Arthralgia/Joint Pain | 55097 |
| Kawasaki Disease | 32 |
| Systemic Inflammatory Response Syndrome | 473 |

The same **adverse event** outcomes have been listed by the **FDA** in their own documents also, which can be found here: https://www.fda.gov/media/143557/download. These are not all of the possible adverse reactions. There have been anecdotal reports of low white blood cell counts also.

The following is a screenshot of the **ingredients** in the **Pfizer**, **Moderna**, and **Johnson and Johnson vaccines**, taken from Appendix C on cdc.gov:

| Description | Pfizer-BioNTech (mRNA) For persons aged 5-11 years (10 µg dose) formulation | Pfizer-BioNTech (mRNA) For persons aged ≥12 years (30 µg dose) formulation | Moderna (mRNA) For persons aged ≥18 years | Janssen (viral vector) For persons aged ≥18 years |
|---|---|---|---|---|
| Active ingredient | Nucleoside-modified mRNA encoding the viral spike (S) glycoprotein of SARS-CoV-2 | Nucleoside-modified mRNA encoding the viral spike (S) glycoprotein of SARS-CoV-2 | Nucleoside-modified mRNA encoding the viral spike (S) glycoprotein of SARS-CoV-2 | Recombinant, replication-incompetent Ad26 vector, encoding a stabilized variant of the SARS-CoV-2 Spike (S) protein |
| Inactive ingredients | 2[(polyethylene glycol (PEG))-2000]-N,N-ditetradecylacetamide | 2[(polyethylene glycol (PEG))-2000]-N,N-ditetradecylacetamide | PEG2000-DMG:1,2-dimyristoyl-rac-glycerol, methoxypolyethylene glycol | Polysorbate-80 |
| | 1,2-distearoyl-sn-glycero-3-phosphocholine | 1,2-distearoyl-sn-glycero-3-phosphocholine | 1,2-distearoyl-sn-glycero-3-phosphocholine | 2-hydroxypropyl-β-cyclodextrin |
| | Cholesterol | Cholesterol | Cholesterol | Citric acid monohydrate |
| | (4-hydroxybutyl)azanediyl)bis(hexane-6,1-diyl)bis(2-hexyldecanoate) | (4-hydroxybutyl)azanediyl)bis(hexane-6,1-diyl)bis(2-hexyldecanoate) | SM-102:heptadecan-9-yl 8-((2-hydroxyethyl) (6-oxo-6-(undecyloxy) hexyl) amino) octanoate | Trisodium citrate dihydrate |
| | Tromethamine | Sodium chloride | Tromethamine | Sodium chloride |
| | Tromethamine hydrochloride | Monobasic potassium phosphate | Tromethamine hydrochloride | Ethanol |
| | Sucrose | Potassium chloride | Acetic acid | |
| | | Dibasic sodium phosphate dihydrate | Sodium acetate | |
| | | Sucrose | Sucrose | |

A number of these ingredients are **synthetic** and may be harmful. In addition, it has been speculated by multiple doctors and researchers, upon examination under microscope, that some or all of these vaccines may possibly contain **graphene oxide** and other unknown materials not listed as ingredients. For more information on graphene oxide, go to https://www.youtube.com/watch?v=cNin-qG1b4o and watch the video by Collin Gow, C.N.C. depicted below:

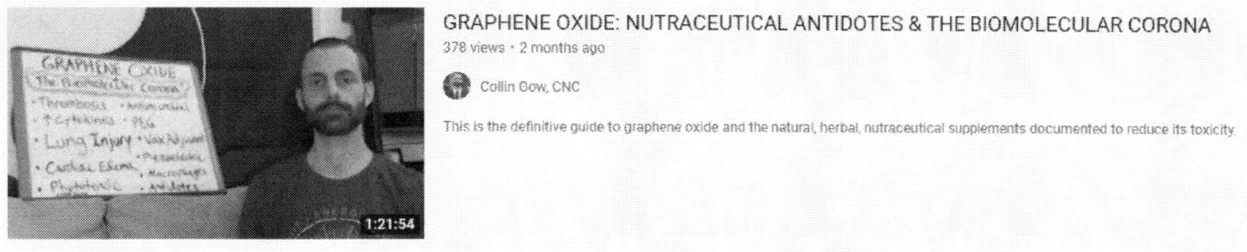


If you or a loved one is suffering from side effects from COVID-19 vaccination, there are remedies you or they may want to consider. **Pick 5 of the following:**

1. **Glutathione or NAC**, 500–1000mg 2x/day on empty stomach to detoxify harmful compounds
2. **Vital Earth Fulvic/Humic Mineral Blend or Shilajit** to detoxify graphene oxide
3. **Chaga**, 2–3g/day with food to boost S.O.D. (antioxidant enzyme), modulate immunity, protect DNA from damage, and repair DNA
4. **Cat's Claw**, 1000mg 2x/day with food to modulate immunity and protect the tissues and organs from damage and inflammation caused by the spike protein being produced in response to the vaccines
5. **Pine Needle Tea or Star Anise Tea**, (high in shikimic acid) 1–2 cups/day to reduce the damage and inflammation from the spike protein
6. **Ginger**, **Garlic**, **Fish Oil**, **Vitamin E**, **Nattokinase**, **Grapeseed Extract**, or very small amount of **Cayenne** to thin the blood and reduce clotting risk
7. **Zinc**, 15mg 2x/day and **Quercetin**, 1000mg 2x/day with food for immunity and allergy
8. **Vitamin D3**, 5,000–10,000 IU/day with food for immunity and allergy
9. **Fennel**, 1000mg 3x/day with meals to reduce damage and inflammation from the spike protein
10. **Curcumin**, 750mg 2x/day to reduce inflammation/cytokines
11. **Magnesium L-Threonate**, **St. John's Wort**, **Gotu Kola** (do not consume if pregnant), **Taurine**, **Choline**, **R-Lipoic Acid**, **Benfothiamine**, **Acetyl-L-Carnitine**, or a **Whole Food B-Complex** for nervous system protection, repair, and/or relaxation
12. **CoQ10**, **Pomegranate Juice**, **Hawthorn**, **Acetyl-L-Carnitine**, **Magnesium Taurate**, **Resveratrol**, **Garlic**, or **Red Wine Extract** for heart health/heart inflammation
13. **Vitamin K1** (ONLY IF THROMBOCYTOPENIA DEVELOPS AND ONLY IN COMBINATION WITH A REMEDY FROM #6 ON THIS LIST)

**Eat a healthy diet** containing high amounts of fruits, vegetables, herbs, spices, nuts, seeds, legumes, mushrooms, onions, garlic, seaweeds, **dark chocolate**, **tomatoes**, underground storage organs (potatoes, sweet potatoes, purple potatoes, yams, yuca, cassava), and squashes. Limit meats & processed foods. Minimal fish, egg yolks, & organ meats is okay (3oz/day).

# Post Virus Recovery

Collin Gow, C.N.C.

1/16/22

When a virus challenges your immune system, your body has to mount and carry out a defense against the attack. This is stressful on your body. It can deplete your reserves, dehydrate you, and cause inflammation. After fighting an infection, you may find yourself feeling fatigued, you may have lost your sense of taste or smell, your hair may be falling out, you may have a cough that won't go away, or you may have difficulty breathing, chest pain, muscle weakness, joint pain, headaches, brain fog, diarrhea, or other symptoms.[1–4] Your lungs, heart, brain, kidneys, and/or other systems may have been damaged. Histopathological findings could be endothelial damage, alveolar damage, pulmonary fibrosis, myocyte injury, hypoxic injury, tubular necrosis, glomerularsclerosis, or other issues.[4] You may be referred to as a "long-hauler" or someone may say that you have "post acute ___________ syndrome". Certain drugs or supplements you took during illness may have given you after-effects as well. Fortunately, you can do something about it. Here are some natural food, supplement, and lifestyle considerations for each indication:

**Fatigue and muscle weakness:** multivitamin, carnitine, and olive leaf[5], rhodiola, schisandra, iron, COQ10, creatine, electrolytes, fruit, plant protein, calcium

**Headaches, joint pain, chest pain:** decaf green tea, resveratrol, cannabinoids, curcumin, and quercetin,[6] andrographis, devils claw, boswellia, msm, magnesium, arjuna, hawthorn, mung bean extract, omega-3s, olive leaf, carnitine

**Dehydration:** electrolyte, kelp, magnesium, hyaluronic acid, spring water, fruits and vegetables, bone broth

**Hair loss/telogen effluvium:** iron, vitamin C, and calories,[7] royal jelly, nettles, horsetail, collagen, bamboo extract

**Loss of smell and taste (anosmia and aguesia):** zinc,[8,9] smell training using rose, eucalyptus, lemon, and clove oils,[10] beta-caryophyllene,[10] raw honey, silver, vitamin A, echinacea, licorice tea, slippery elm lozenges, oral probiotic, & nerve remedies[10] such as lion's mane, choline, and a whole food b-complex

**Brain fog:** lion's mane, blue green algae, choline, serine, iodine, coconut oil, sage, berries

**Chronic cough/lung damage/sensory neuropathic cough:** EPA + GLA,[11] NAC, vitamin A, licorice, black seed oil, boswellia, silica, mullein, chickweed, horehound, coltsfoot, marshmallow, peppermint, eucalyptus, pleurisy, and nerve remedies[12] such as GABA, cannabinoids, taurine, lion's mane

**Difficulty breathing:** oxygen cans, iron, chlorophyll or copper, vitamin C, cordyceps, peppermint, carnitine, rhodiola, yohimbe, butcher's broom, Liquid Light, boswellia, mullein, chickweed, horehound, coltsfoot, marshmallow, licorice, pleurisy, NAC, Oxypower, vitamin A, citrus fruits, sea salt, spring water

**Diarrhea:** psyllium, prebiotic, probiotic, saccharomyces boulardii, red raspberry leaf, boswellia, vitamin A

**Immune system support/other:** cat's claw, fennel, pine needle tea, star anise, probiotic

**All the above:** Myers cocktail I.V.

**Diet:** eat a nearly plant-based diet,[13] with high amounts of fruits and vegetables, consume citrus, kelp, sea salt, plant protein, small amounts of liver (high in vitamin A), iron rich foods such as molasses, liver, kale, spinach, and legumes and drink spring water

**Lifestyle:** focus on sleep and rest before jumping back into your normal lifestyle and exercise routine. Reduce your work and stress load. Once all your symptoms are gone, choose low intensity, light forms of physical movement. Take a walk in nature. Practice qi gong or deep breathing exercises.

This is article was not an attempt to treat, diagnose, prevent, or cure any disease or condition. Talk to your doctor before making any changes.

References:


1. Pavli A, Theodoridou M, Maltezou HC. Post-COVID Syndrome: Incidence, Clinical Spectrum, and Challenges for Primary Healthcare Professionals. Arch Med Res. 2021 Aug;52(6):575-581. doi: 10.1016/j.arcmed.2021.03.010. Epub 2021 May 4. PMID: 33962805; PMCID: PMC8093949.
2. Lopez-Leon S, Wegman-Ostrosky T, Perelman C, Sepulveda R, Rebolledo PA, Cuapio A, Villapol S. More than 50 long-term effects of COVID-19: a systematic review and meta-analysis. Sci Rep. 2021 Aug 9;11(1):16144. doi: 10.1038/s41598-021-95565-8. PMID: 34373540; PMCID: PMC8352980.
3. Cereda E, Clavé P, Collins PF, Holdoway A, Wischmeyer PE. Recovery Focused Nutritional Therapy across the Continuum of Care: Learning from COVID-19. Nutrients. 2021 Sep 21;13(9):3293. doi: 10.3390/nu13093293. PMID: 34579171; PMCID: PMC8472175.
4. Chippa V, Aleem A, Anjum F. Post Acute Coronavirus (COVID-19) Syndrome. [Updated 2021 Oct 1]. In: StatPearls [Internet]. Treasure Island (FL): StatPearls Publishing; 2021 Jan-. Available from: https://www.ncbi.nlm.nih.gov/books/NBK570608/
5. Naureen Z, Dautaj A, Nodari S, Fioretti F, Dhuli K, Anpilogov K, Lorusso L, Paolacci S, Michelini S, Guda T, Kallazi M, Bertelli M. Proposal of a food supplement for the management of post-COVID syndrome. Eur Rev Med Pharmacol Sci. 2021 Dec;25(1 Suppl):67-73. doi: 10.26355/eurrev_202112_27335. PMID: 34890036.
6. Giovinazzo G, Gerardi C, Uberti-Foppa C, Lopalco L. Can Natural Polyphenols Help in Reducing Cytokine Storm in COVID-19 Patients? Molecules. 2020 Dec 12;25(24):5888. doi: 10.3390/molecules25245888. PMID: 33322757; PMCID: PMC7763290.
7. Almohanna HM, Ahmed AA, Tsatalis JP, Tosti A. The Role of Vitamins and Minerals in Hair Loss: A Review. Dermatol Ther (Heidelb). 2019 Mar;9(1):51-70. doi: 10.1007/s13555-018-0278-6. Epub 2018 Dec 13. PMID: 30547302; PMCID: PMC6380979.
8. Propper RE. Smell/Taste alteration in COVID-19 may reflect zinc deficiency. J Clin Biochem Nutr. 2021 Jan;68(1):3. doi: 10.3164/jcbn.20-177. Epub 2021 Jan 1. PMID: 33536704; PMCID: PMC7844651.

9. Hummel T, Landis BN, Hüttenbrink KB. Smell and taste disorders. GMS Curr Top Otorhinolaryngol Head Neck Surg. 2011;10:Doc04. doi: 10.3205/cto000077. Epub 2012 Apr 26. PMID: 22558054; PMCID: PMC3341581.
10. Koyama S, Kondo K, Ueha R, Kashiwadani H, Heinbockel T. Possible Use of Phytochemicals for Recovery from COVID-19-Induced Anosmia and Ageusia. Int J Mol Sci. 2021 Aug 18;22(16):8912. doi: 10.3390/ijms22168912. PMID: 34445619; PMCID: PMC8396277.
11. Pacht ER, DeMichele SJ, Nelson JL, Hart J, Wennberg AK, Gadek JE. Enteral nutrition with eicosapentaenoic acid, gamma-linolenic acid, and antioxidants reduces alveolar inflammatory mediators and protein influx in patients with acute respiratory distress syndrome. Crit Care Med. 2003 Feb;31(2):491-500. doi: 10.1097/01.CCM.0000049952.96496.3E. PMID: 12576957.
12. Laryngopedia. (2021, March 3). *Still Coughing After COVID? | Sensory Neuropathic Cough (SNC)*. YouTube. Retrieved January 16, 2022, from https://www.youtube.com/watch?v=MWxbFiiQPi0
13. Storz MA. Lifestyle Adjustments in Long-COVID Management: Potential Benefits of Plant-Based Diets. Curr Nutr Rep. 2021 Dec;10(4):352-363. doi: 10.1007/s13668-021-00369-x. Epub 2021 Sep 10. PMID: 34506003; PMCID: PMC8429479.

# Should I Vaccinate My Child for COVID-19
# or
# Support My Child's Natural Immunity?

Collin Gow, C.N.C.
11/19/2021

About 40 doses of vaccines are already recommended by age 11 by the CDC on their immunization schedule. That information can be found here: https://www.cdc.gov/vaccines/schedules/hcp/imz/child-adolescent.html. Adding more "vaccines" to that schedule may not be the greatest idea, especially when you consider the ingredients in vaccines.

**What are the ingredients in vaccines?**

- Human fetal lung fibroblast cells
- Protein from human blood
- Monkey kidney cells
- Protein from cow blood
- Mutant of diptheria toxin
- Adhesive polymers
- Milk sugar
- Plasticizer chemicals (phthalates)
- Artificial dyes
- Acetone
- Aluminum
- Casein
- Mercury
- Sucrose
- Sugar alcohols
- Formaldehyde
- Amino alcohols
- Polysorbate 80
- Antibiotics
- Disinfectants
- Genetically engineered ingredients
- Bile acids
- Polyethylene glycol
- Ammonia
- Live viruses

https://www.cdc.gov/vaccines/pubs/pinkbook/downloads/appendices/b/excipient-table-2.pdf
http://www.vaccinesafety.edu/components-Excipients.htm

**What are the ingredients in the Pfizer-Biontech COVID-19 "vaccine" for ages 5–11?**

mRNA, lipids ((4-hydroxybutyl)azanediyl)bis(hexane-6,1-diyl)bis(2-hexyldecanoate), 2 [(polyethylene glycol)-2000]-N,N-ditetradecylacetamide, 1,2-Distearoyl-sn-glycero-3-phosphocholine, and cholesterol), tromethamine, tromethamine hydrochloride, sucrose, and sodium chloride.
https://www.fda.gov/media/153717/download

**What side effects to COVID-19 vaccines have been reported?**

Guillaine Barre, Acute Disseminated Encephalomyelitis, Transverse Myelitis, Encephalitis, Convulsions/Seizures, Stroke, Narcolepsy, Cataplexy, Anaphylaxis, Acute Myocardial Infarction (Heart Attack), Myocarditis/Pericarditis, Autoimmune Disease, Other Acute Demyelinating Diseases, Pregnancy and birth outcomes (Miscarriages), Other Allergic Reactions, Thrombocytopenia, Disseminated Intravascular Coagulation, Venous Thromboembolism, Arthritis and Arthralgia/Joint Pain, Kawasaki Disease, Systemic Inflammatory Response Syndrome, Death. vaers.hhs.gov
https://www.fda.gov/media/143557/download

**Are vaccines safe and effective?**

Considering the ingredients and side effects above, the answer has to be no, regardless of the fact that some have undergone phase 1, 2, and 3 clinical trials (the Pfizer-Biontech "vaccine" has). At least half of the scientific literature in general these days may be untrue due to major conflicts of interest and other problems, (Gyles et al.). However, the CDC and other governing bodies claim that the COVID vaccines are safe and effective. But what does "safe and effective" actually mean? "Safe" means that a vaccine has undergone clinical trials, FDA review, and the benefits are said to outweigh the risks. "Effective" means that the vaccine has undergone clinical trials, been reviewed by the FDA, elicits an antibody response, and that it doesn't lose much effectiveness through storage and delivery.
https://www.cdc.gov/flu/vaccines-work/effectivenessqa.htm
https://www.cdc.gov/vaccinesafety/research/index.html
https://www.cdc.gov/vaccines/parents/infographics/journey-of-child-vaccine.html

**What is the chance that my child will die of COVID-19?**

There have been 94 COVID-19 deaths from January 1, 2020 to October 16, 2021 in children ages 5–11 in the U.S.. https://www.cdc.gov/vaccines/acip/meetings/downloads/slides-2021-11-2-3/03-COVID-Jefferson-508.pdf There were 24.4 million children aged 6-11 alive in the United States as of 2019.
https://www.statista.com/statistics/457786/number-of-children-in-the-us-by-age/
That is a 1 in 259,574 chance that a child between age 6-11 would die of COVID-19.

**Can you sue a vaccine manufacturer if your child is damaged by a vaccine?**

No. That is why the governmental National Vaccine Injury Compensation Program exists.

**If your child has been injured by a vaccine and you are seeking compensation, go here:**
https://www.hrsa.gov/vaccine-compensation/index.html
**For COVID vaccine injury go here:**
https://www.hrsa.gov/cicp

**Is the Pfizer-Biontech COVID-19 vaccine FDA approved for children ages 5–11?**

No. It has been authorized for emergency use only. It has not been FDA "approved". "Under an EUA [Emergency Use Authorization], FDA may allow the use of unapproved medical products, or unapproved uses of approved medical products in an emergency to diagnose, treat, or prevent serious or life-threatening diseases or conditions when certain statutory criteria have been met, including that there are no adequate, approved, and available alternatives. Taking into consideration input from the FDA, manufacturers decide whether and when to submit an EUA request to FDA."
https://www.fda.gov/news-events/press-announcements/fda-authorizes-pfizer-biontech-covid-19-vaccine-emergency-use-children-5-through-11-years-age

**Has the Pfizer-Biontech COVID-19 vaccine been studied in children?**

It has been studied for safety in approximately 3,100 children age 5 through 11 and "no serious side effects have been detected". Obviously, the FDA's definition of "side effects" is a pretty loose definition. "In addition, the vaccine was found to be 90.7% effective in preventing COVID-19 in children 5 through 11." https://www.fda.gov/news-events/press-announcements/fda-authorizes-pfizer-biontech-covid-19-vaccine-emergency-use-children-5-through-11-years-age

**Can you trust the FDA, the CDC, and Pfizer?**

The FDA receives 45% of its annual budget from the pharmaceutical industry. Bill Gates gave the CDC

$1 million in 2003, $30 million in 2013/14, and he gave a combined $20 million to groups including the CDC in 2020 to combat COVID-19. This exorbitant private funding of a "public" agency creates conflicts of interest. Pfizer agreed to pay the largest criminal fine in U.S. history in 2009 at $2.3 billion for fraudulent marketing. You tell me.

**If my child gets "vaccinated" for COVID-19 can he or she still get COVID-19?**
Yes. https://www.cdc.gov/coronavirus/2019-ncov/vaccines/effectiveness/why-measure-effectiveness/breakthrough-cases.html#:~:text=Most%20people%20who%20get%20COVID,%E2%80%9Cbreakthrough%20infection.%E2%80%9D

**Why do we have an immune system?**
To identify, neutralize, protect, and eliminate threats from other species or pathogenic microbes. The body has neutrophils, lymphocytes, monocytes, basophils, eosinophils, dendritic cells, macrophages, natural killer cells, mast cells, and other systems to deal with foreign invaders. Consider supporting your child's natural immunity for a robust antiviral response.

# How Can I Support My Child's Natural Immunity?

**Supplements**

1. Baker's yeast or Nutritional Yeast or Beta-Glucans (Saccharomyces cerevisiae) have been shown to reduce the risk of respiratory infections in children, (Jesenak, Milos et al.)
2. Zinc, 5–10mg/day
3. Vitamin D3, 1,000–3,000IU/day
4. Probiotic, 1 Billion–5 Billion/day
5. Elderberry Syrup or Gummies
6. Lemon Balm Tincture
7. Echinacea/Astragalus Tincture
8. Multivitamin
9. Colostrum
10. Whole Food Vitamin C

**Foods**

Consume a healthy diet of whole fruits, vegetables, herbs, spices, underground storage organs (potatoes, sweet potatoes, purple potatoes), squashes, legumes, mushrooms, garlic, onions, ginger, peppers, citrus fruits, fermented foods, manuka honey, nutritional yeast, seaweed, pumpkin seeds, and brazil nuts. Limit refined and processed foods. Minimal amounts of fish, egg yolks, & organ meats is okay.

# About the Author

Available for purchase @ www.collingowcnc.wixsite.com/collingowcnc

# Gut Problems?

**Leaky gut? IBS? IBD? UC? Diverticulosis? Constipation? Food Sensitivities? Autoimmunity? Overweight?**

*** Powerful Postbiotic! ***

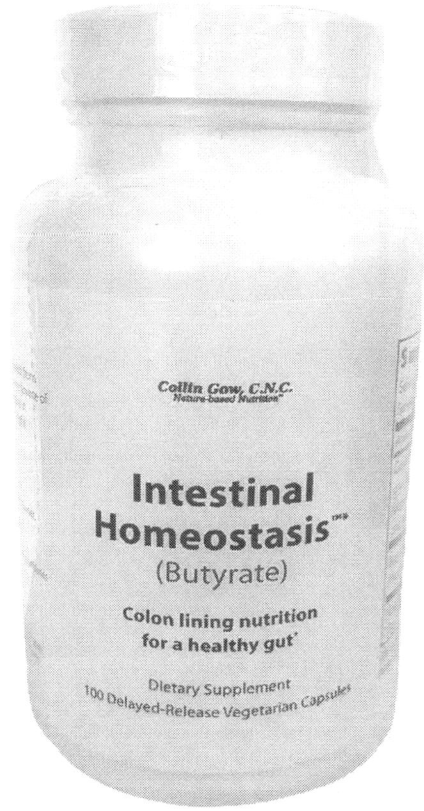


*** Fuel For Colon Cells! ***

**Over 40 clinically proven beneficial effects of butyrate can't be wrong!**

**↑Tight Junctions* ↑Gut Barrier Integrity* ↓Inflammation***
**↑Beneficial Bacteria* ↑Absorption* ↓Appetite* •Antioxidant***
**•Antitumor* •Modulates G.I. Motility*& Innate Immunity***
**•Supports Normal Intestinal PH*& Intestinal Mucosa Homeostasis***
**↓Insulin Resistance* ↑Metabolism* ↑Antimicrobial Peptides***
**•Modulates Neuronal Excitability* ↑Glutathione* ↓Endotoxins***

References and Purchase @ www.collingowcnc.wixsite.com/naturevorenutrition/supplements

*These statements have not been evaluated by the FDA. This product is not intended to treat, diagnose, prevent, or cure any disease or condition.

Available for purchase @ www.collingowcnc.wixsite.com/collingowcnc

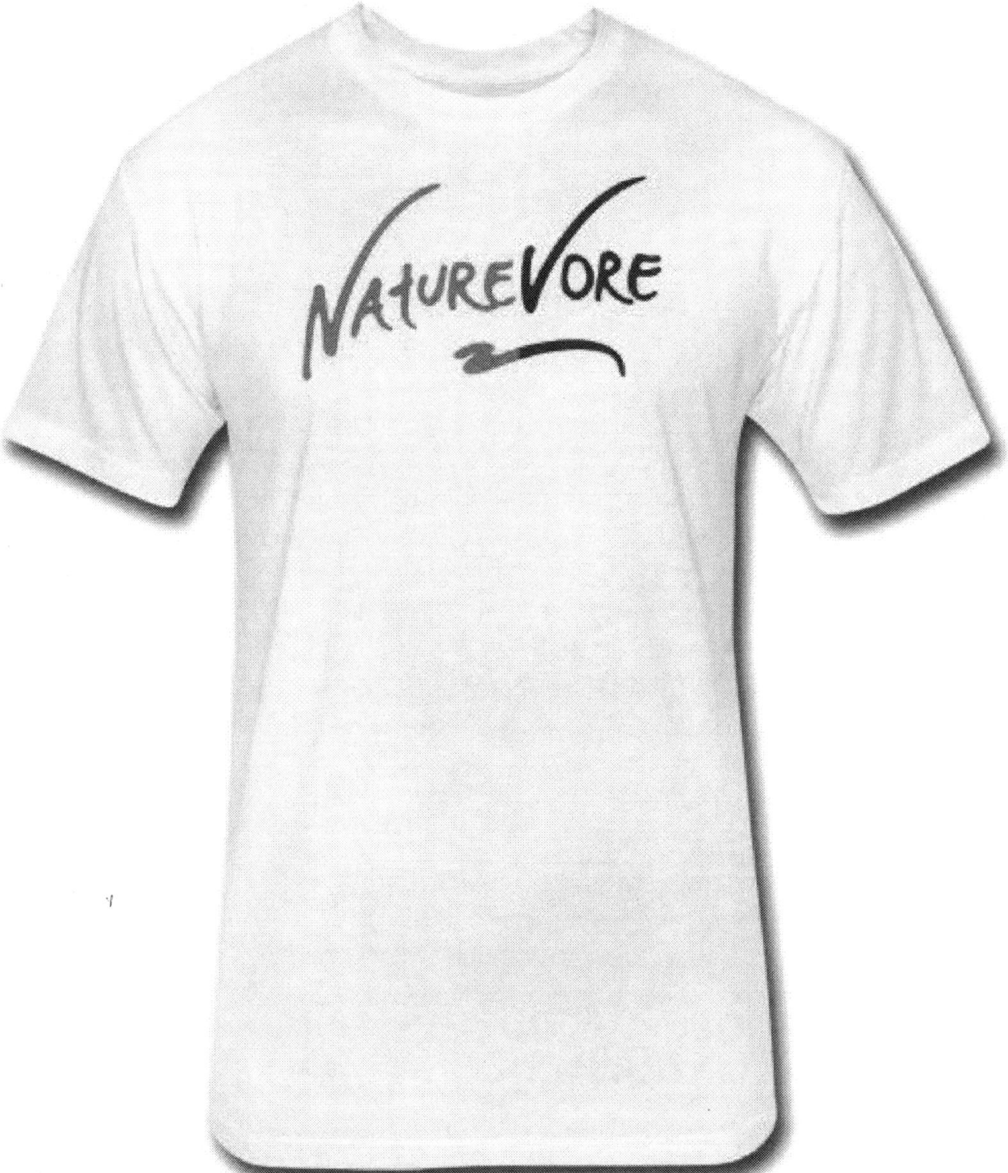

Available for purchase @ www.collingowcnc.wixsite.com/collingowcnc

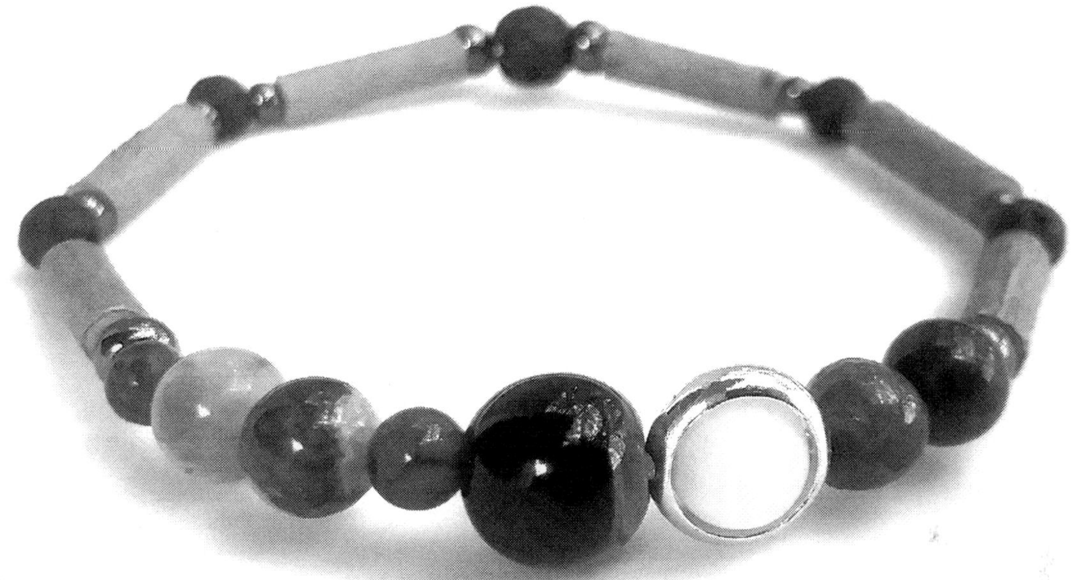

https://us.fullscript.com/welcome/collingowcnc

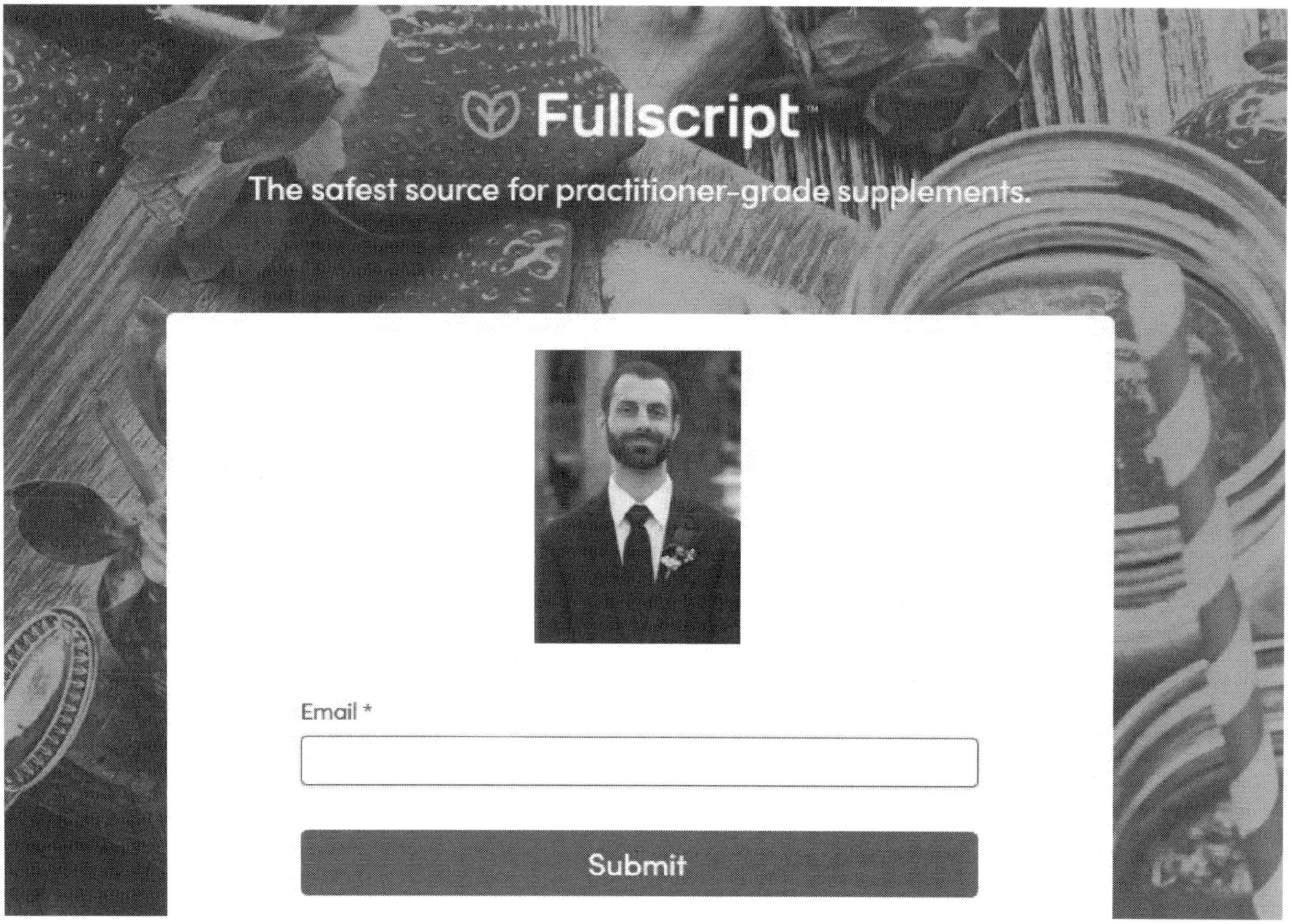

Available for purchase @ www.collingowcnc.wixsite.com/collingowcnc

This educational, eye-opening volume contains thoroughly investigated and referenced complementary and alternative remedies for bolstering immunity in the face of COVID-19 and other viral infections, recovering from Long COVID, and detoxifying and healing after vaccination. Also present are articles/information on vaccine ingredients and side effects, graphene oxide, and face masks. Are you having lingering symptoms such as loss of taste or smell, fatigue, chronic cough, difficulty breathing, hair loss, diarrhea, brain fog, joint pain, headaches, chest pain, or dehydration? This book covers all that. There are food, supplement, and lifestyle recommendations on each topic. Dashes of "conspiracy" are sprinkled into the volume here and there too. Collin calls out the corrupt, conflict-of-interest-laden elites and captured agencies that are supposedly looking out for our health. Anthony Fauci, Bill Gates, the CDC, the WHO, the UN, and others make appearances. Event 201, vaccine patents, 5G, and Agenda 21/2030 are discussed. However, this is a serious book, by a real practitioner, not woo woo flim-flam. It is filled with data from scientific publications and medical journal studies to back up the time-tested natural compounds it mentions. This is your no-nonsense guide to surviving COVID-19, Post COVID syndrome, mask wearing, and vaccination.

If you're looking for the most complete, detailed, well-researched, well-documented, clinical book out there on holistic, nutritional, nutraceutical approaches to immunity, pandemics, plandemics, viruses, vaccines, COVID-19, Long COVID, masks, graphene oxide, and more, then look no further. This is it. If you're interested in health freedom and you dislike Big Pharma tyranny and allopathic, medical authoritarianism, then buy this book!

Collin Gow, C.N.C. is a certified nutritional consultant and author of 4 books. He has been researching for 21 years and been a practitioner in the fields of health and nutrition for 13 years at the time of first publication of this book. Collin has also appeared on radio, TV, Youtube, and in print. He has a holistic, scientific, personal, evidence-based, and nature-based approach to health and healing and he has helped hundreds of thousands of people get well.

Be sure to check out Collin's other books for sale on Amazon or go to collingowcnc.wixsite.com/collingowcnc

**Collin Gow, C.N.C.**
*Nature-based Nutrition™*

$22.99
ISBN 978-0-578-36514-5
52299>
9 780578 365145

# Clinical Nutrition, COVID-19, and Long COVID

## (+ Vaccines, Graphene Oxide, Masks, and Other Viruses)

### Holistic, Scientific, Natural, Herbal, Nature-Based Immunity and Recovery

**Collin Gow, C.N.C.**

Available for purchase @ www.collingowcnc.wixsite.com/collingowcnc

Collin Gow, C.N.C. is a certified nutritional consultant who has been working in the fields of health and nutrition for 12 years and researching for over 20 years at the time of first publication of this book. Appearing on Youtube, radio, TV, and in print, Collin does it all. As someone who has gone through his own health challenges, he has gained not only book learning, but crucial experiential knowledge and insights about natural foods and supplements so often lacking in conventional medicine. Collin has a holistic, scientific, personalized, and nature-based approach to health and healing and he has helped hundreds of thousands of people get well.

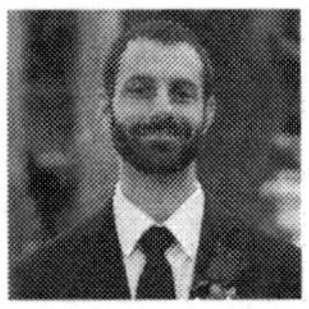

The present volume is packed with holistic, nutritional wisdom and scientific evidence gleaned from a myriad of medical journal studies. It covers subjects such as hormones, weight loss, superfoods, energy, sleep, gut, heart, thyroid, and immune health, as well as abnormal cell growth, viruses, mold, vaccines, specialty supplements, and more. It includes food, supplement, and lifestyle recommendations on each topic. Collin is well-versed in the fields of natural, complementary, lifestyle, and alternative medicine, naturopathy, holistic nutrition, herbalism, homeopathy, Chinese medicine, Ayurveda, biochemistry, food science, dietetics, epigenetics, anatomy, physiology, microbiology, ethnomedicine, zoopharmacognosy, evolutionary nutrition, comparative nutrition, philosophy of nutrition, autoimmunity, candida, veganism, plant-based diets, blood-type diets, lectin avoidance diets, paleo, keto, GAPS, FODMAP, food combining, and more!

$28.99
ISBN 978-0-578-88569-8
52899>
9 780578 885698

**Collin Gow, C.N.C.**
*Nature-based Nutrition™*

# Collin Gow, C.N.C.

## Collected Works on Health and Nutrition, Volume 1 (2017-2020)

Collin Gow, C.N.C.

Available for purchase @ www.collingowcnc.wixsite.com/collingowcnc

Collin Gow, C.N.C. is a renaissance man. Before focusing his career on health, nutrition, and writing, Collin spent 10 years as a teenager and young adult passionately pursuing art. Creating has always made him feel better than anything else in life. This book is an assemblage of the artworks done by Collin throughout those creative years and beyond. Collin's art encompasses a multitude of styles, including crummy, outsider, sketchy, primitive, ignorant, shitty, scratch, gonzo, street, cartoon, abstract, graphic, graffiti, pop, ball-point pen, rollerball, pencil, stencil, and portrait art. Many mediums have been used by Collin as well and can be seen in this book. Collin's art is generally aphoristic, inspirational, and rebellious, often with meaningful quotations appearing in it, and it covers subjects such as philosophy, genius, greatness, art, happiness, love, relationships, studying, music, movies, kids, skateboarding, holistic health, nutrition, fitness,

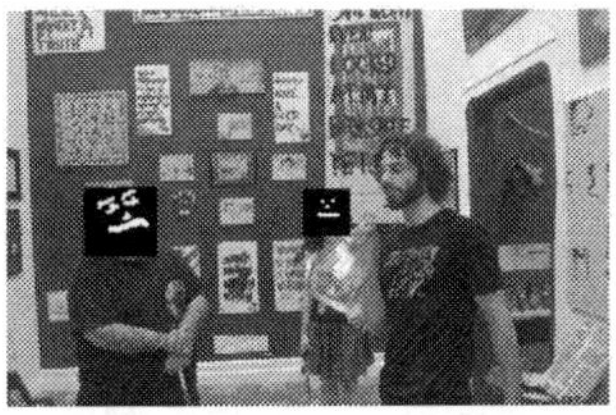

nature, naturevore, naturotheology, astrology, astrotheology, numerology, science, math, sacred geometry, quantum physics, psychology, spirituality, ancient knowledge, and more. Similarities could be pointed out between Collin's art and the art of Daniel Johnston, Mark Gonzales, Shel Silverstein, Ralph Steadman, Jean-Michel Basquiat, and/or Tai Taeoalii. Other heroes or influences include Picasso, Kandinsky, Michelangelo, Arnold Schwarzenegger, Ian Gow, James Rise, Andy Warhol, Chuck Close, Leonardo Da Vinci, Jackson Pollock, and Salvador Dali. Collin pales in comparison to these greats, but he is confident that the shear amount, uniqueness, profundity, depth, and meaningfulness of his art, stacked alongside his myriad other accomplishments, will be held in high regard by those who come after him. Enjoy his beautiful, deep, whacky, thoughtful, unique, mind-expanding, shitty, quirky, inspirational, and versatile creations.

$35.99
ISBN 978-0-578-94622-1
53599>

# Collin Gow, C.N.C.

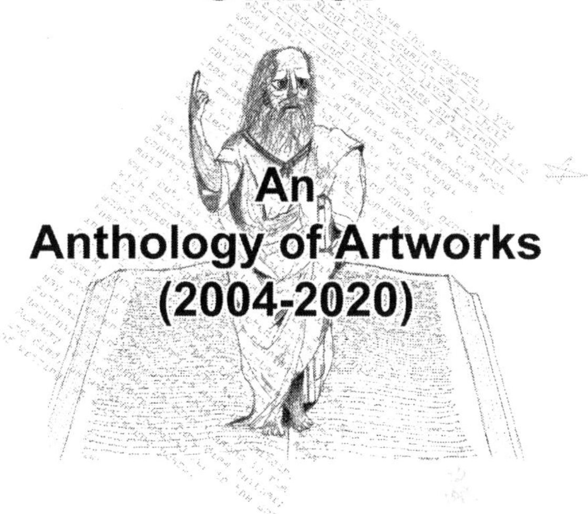

## An Anthology of Artworks (2004-2020)

Collin Gow, C.N.C.

Available for purchase @ www.collingowcnc.wixsite.com/collingowcnc

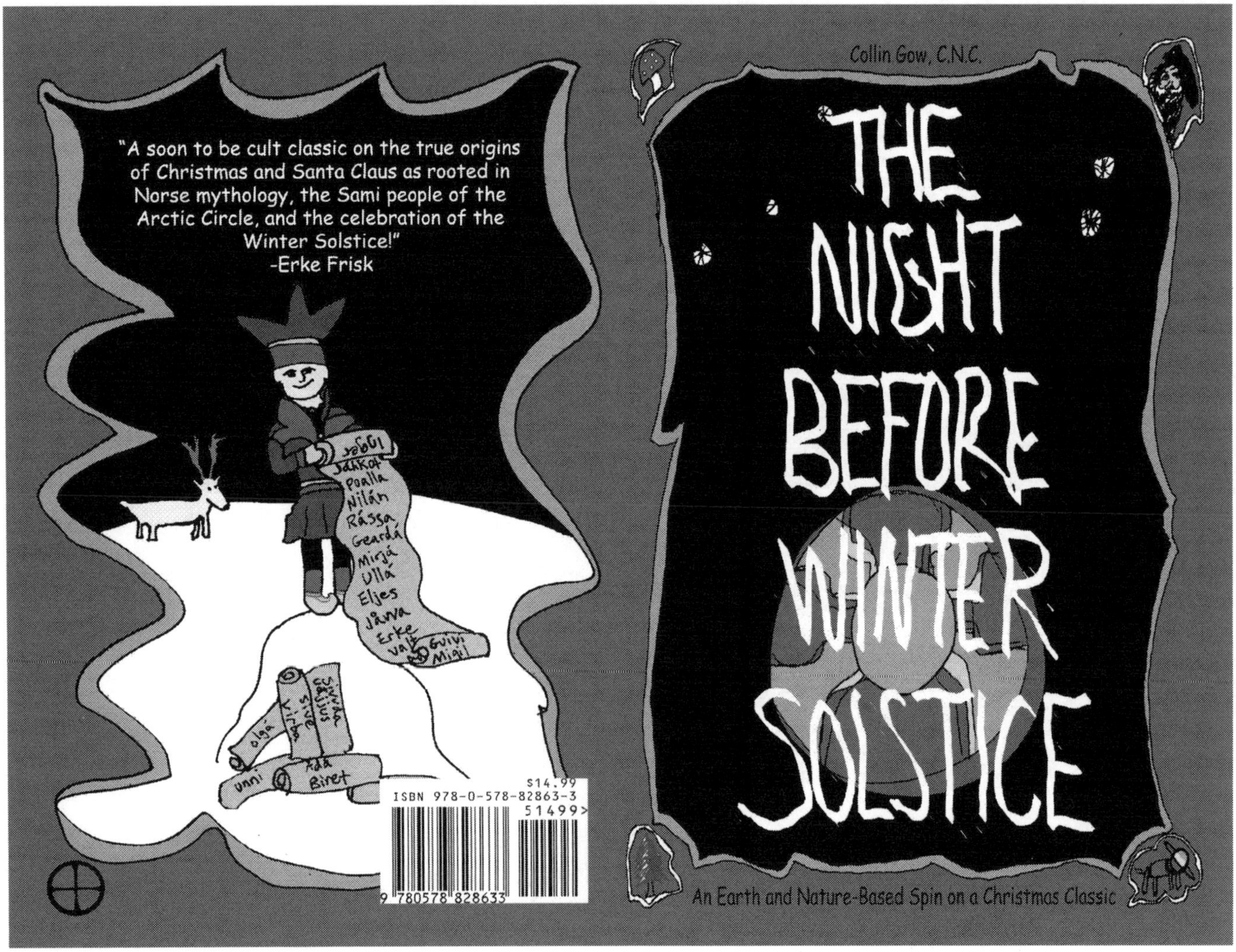

# Collin Gow, C.N.C.

is an author, certified nutritional consultant, naturevore, naturotheologist, and father.

**Collin's Websites**

www.collingowcnc.wixsite.com/collingowcnc
www.collingowcnc.wixsite.com/naturevorenutrition
www.collingowcnc.wixsite.com/naturotheology
www.collingowcnc.com (under construction as of 3/14/2022)
www.naturevorenutrition.com (under construction as of 3/14/2022)
www.naturotheology.org (under construction as of 3/14/2022)

**Collin's Other Books**

- *Clinical Nutrition, COVID-19, and Long COVID (+ Vaccines, Graphene Oxide, Masks, and Other Viruses): Holistic, Scientific, Natural, Herbal, Nature-Based Immunity and Recovery*

- *Collin Gow, C.N.C.: Collected Works on Health and Nutrition, Volume 1 (2017–2020)*

- *The Night Before Winter Solstice: An Earth and Nature-Based Spin on a Christmas Classic*

- *Collin Gow, C.N.C.: An Anthology of Artworks (2004–2020)*

All available for purchase on Amazon @
https://www.amazon.com/Collin-Gow-C.N.C./e/B08RWMRYQR
%3Fref=dbs_a_mng_rwt_scns_share

Made in United States
Orlando, FL
04 November 2026

90206055R00070